1000 mLs of Truth

The Deposition of Stanley Plotkin

The following is the transcript for the deposition of Stanley Plotkin in January 2018:

MS. NIEUSMA: I'm going to ask that everybody speak up. You're all coming across a little soft other than Maureen. She's doing fine.

VIDEO OPERATOR: This is the start of media labeled number one of the video-recorded deposition of Dr. Stanley Plotkin in the matter of Lori Matheson, formerly known as Lori Ann Schmitt, versus Michael Schmitt, filed in the State of Michigan, Circuit Court, County of Oakland, Family Division. This deposition is being held at 5833 Lower York Road in New Hope, Pennsylvania, on January 11, 2018.

Counsel, please introduce yourselves for the record.

MR. SIRI: Aaron Siri, co-counsel on behalf of plaintiff.

MS. RUBY: Amy Ruby, on behalf -- co-counsel on behalf of plaintiff.

MS. NIEUSMA: Laura Nieusma, counsel for defendant, Michael Schmitt.

VIDEO OPERATOR: The court reporter will now swear in the witness.

-- -

STANLEY PLOTKIN, M.D., having been first duly sworn to tell the truth, was examined and testified as follows:

-- - EXAMINATION

BY MR. SIRI:

Q: Good morning, Dr. Plotkin.

MS. RUBY: Can we just make a record under this...

MR. SIRI: I would just like to clarify that this is being recorded by a video deposition pursuant to MCR 2.315.

BY MR. SIRI:

Q: Good morning. Can you please state your full name for the record.

A: Stanley A. Plotkin.

Q: Dr. Plotkin, have you been deposed before?

A: A long time ago. Many years ago.

Q: In what matter was that?

A: Oh, it had to do with an abortion done because of congenital rubella.

Q: What year approximately?

A: The 1960s.

Q: And what was your testimony about?

A: My testimony was about the abnormalities that occur in infants of women born -- that is, infants of women who have congenital, who have rubella during pregnancy and whose fetuses are frequently affected with considerable congenital abnormalities.

Q: From rubella?

A: From rubella.

Q: Did that involve a vaccine?

A: I, at the time I was developing a vaccine against rubella; yes.

Q: Have you been deposed in any other case?

A: Not that I can recall, no.

Q: Have you ever been an expert witness in any lawsuit other than this one?

A: Again, not for many years. I believe I did a couple of those cases in the '60s, but I have avoided depositions since then.

Q: Why is that?

A: Because I consider that they seldom bring out all the facts, but I'm willing to help in this case.

Q: I'm going to go over a few rules with you for this deposition.

A: Mm-hmm.

Q: The court reporter has placed you under oath. Same as a court of law, you're testifying under penalty of perjury.

A: Mm-hmm.

Q: The court reporter's making a record and will take down the questions that I ask and the answers that you provide.

A: Mm-hmm.

Q: If you don't understand a question, let me know before answering. Okay? The court reporter can't take down nods. That's another rule. So if you -.

A: Yes.

Q: Anytime you want to vocalize, please wait until I complete asking a given question, even if you think you know the answer, so that we have a complete record, please. As I -- don't speculate. If you don't know the answer, then so state. But you should provide your best recollection, even if it's vague or partial. Okay?

A: Yes.

Q: Are you taking any medications or are under the influence of any substance that might affect your ability to testify today?

A: I don't think so, no.

Q: Is that no?

A: No.

Q: Okay. Did you discuss this deposition with anyone?

A: Actually, no. I've had some conversations with Laura Nieusma, but not about the substance of my testimony.

Q: Before today, did you have any discussions with anyone related to this deposition?

A: No. Actually, I know very little about the issue here. I understand that there's a disagreement between parents, but that's all I really know.

Q: And you haven't discussed this lawsuit with anyone apart from opposing counsel?

A: No.

Q: How did you first learn about this lawsuit?

A: It was from a lady by the name of Karen Ernst, who was the head of an organization called Voices for Vaccines, which is a group of laypeople who are favorable to vaccination. And she had heard from the father, I believe, who was looking for experts to testify on his behalf.

Q: So you discussed this lawsuit with her?

A: Not really discussed the lawsuit. She referred me to the father, and I sent an email saying that I would be willing to testify. I have not talked to the father. I've never met the father. So I, everything has happened secondhand, so to speak.

Q: And it was Karen Ernst who asked you to be an expert in this case?

A: She asked me if I would be willing, yes.

Q: How many discussions have you had with her?

A: No discussions.

Q: About this case.

A: About this case, simply had an email exchange asking me to do it.

Q: I'm going to request a copy of that email chain, okay, Dr. Plotkin?

A: If I can find it, I'll be glad to send it to you.

Q: Thank you. So before today, other than speaking with opposing counsel and an email communication with Karen Ernst, you have not discussed this lawsuit, this deposition, or the role that you'd be playing here today with anybody else; is that right?

A: I've had an email exchange with Paul Offit, Dr. Paul Offit, who is actually a former student of mine.

Q: Who is Dr. Offit?

A: Dr. Offit is a pediatrician at the Children's Hospital of Philadelphia .

Q: What did you discuss with Dr. Offit?

A: I discussed with him the issues or the possible issues about refusal to vaccinate.

Q: What was the substance of those discussions?

A: The substance basically concerned what arguments are often used to oppose vaccination.

Q: What are those arguments?

A: The arguments generally are that vaccines can cause reactions and that the reactions are worse than the disease.

Q: And what did Dr. Offit have to say about that?

A: Well, he pointed out, of course -- and he's the author of a chapter in my Vaccines book -.that the opposite is true, that the disease is worse than the reactions to the vaccines.

Q: Do you have peer-reviewed science to support that statement?

A: Do I have what?

Q: Peer-reviewed science to support that statement?

A: Yes, of course.

Q: Would you be willing to provide that science?

A: Well, the science is in the chapter in my textbook. But there are innumerable references, some of which I have, but I can certainly provide you with a list of references in the chapter.

Q: Great. Have you reviewed any documents to prepare for this deposition?

A: You know, I've looked at the web. I don't usually do that, but I've looked at the web, some of the anti-vaccination websites.

Q: Which of those sites did you look at?

A: Oh, gosh. I can't give you the names. I've just sort of scanned through a number of them.

Q: Do you remember the names of any of them?

A: Let's see.

MS. NIEUSMA: Dr. Plotkin, just to be clear, if you don't remember something, just say you don't remember and you can move on from there.

THE WITNESS: Yeah. Well, here's one called VaxTruth: Everything you ever needed to know about medical exemptions to vaccination but didn't know to ask. There are a couple of others that I looked at, many of which were appalling.

BY MR. SIRI:

Q: Why do you believe they're appalling?

A: Because they're ignorant of the facts, exaggerations, half-truths, or even misconceptions.

Q: VaxTruth, does that website, is that a website that catalogs personal stories of families who believe their child was injured by vaccines?

A: You know, I did not -- what shall I say? -- read these word for word. I imagine that that's the case, but I couldn't tell you specifically about which website says what.

Q: But you found VaxTruth appalling?

A: Yes.

Q: Other than reviewing the, what you refer to as anti-vax or websites, did you review any other documents to prepare for this deposition?

A: Yes. I looked at a number of vaccine safety studies, which, again, are referenced in the vaccine safety chapter.

Q: And apart from that, anything else?

A: No.

Q: Have you been provided any documents related to this lawsuit?

A: To whom?

Q: Have you, Dr. Plotkin, been provided any documents relating to this lawsuit specifically?

A: No, I have not.

Q: Have you reviewed any medical records related to this case?

A: Medical records? No.

Q: Have you done anything other than what we've already discussed to prepare for this deposition today?

A: No. Basically, no.

Q: Have you discussed the child at issue in this case?

A: No.

Q: So you don't know anything specific about the child at issue in this case, correct?

A: I do not.

Q: You don't know anything about her medical history, correct?

A: Correct.

Q: And you don't know anything about her family's medical history, correct?

A: Correct.

Q: Have you been on any trips in the last year?

A: Many.

Q: Where to?

A: Several trips to Europe, to France, to Germany. Let's see. Have I been to Asia in the last year? Yes. I've been to Japan. Basically, I mean, of course, many trips in the United States, England.

Q: How many times -.

A: At least a dozen trips.

Q: At least a dozen. How many times were you in France in the last year?

A: Oh, gosh. Twice, I think.

Q: Germany?

A: Once.

Q: England?

A: Once.

Q: These are all separate trips?

A: Yes.

Q: In which you got on a plane from the United States, flew there, flew back?

A: Yes.

Q: Japan, how many times?

A: Once.

Q: How many times to other countries outside of U.S.?

A: I've probably had about a dozen trips altogether. If I known that you were interested, I would have brought my calendar.

Q: How about trips in the United States that required you to get on a plane, how many of those would you say in the last year?

A: Mainly to California. A lot of trips to Washington. Boston.

Q: California, Washington. Same city in California each time or different?

A: No. San Francisco, San Diego.

Q: What were the purpose of most of these trips?

A: Attend meetings, scientific meetings.

Q: Were any of them related to companies developing vaccines?

A: Oh, yes.

Q: Would you say most of them were?

A: Most of them? Probably about half of them.

Q: Do you have any, do you have any trips planned for 2018?

A: Yes.

Q: Where to?

A: I'll be going to India next month and, however, I'm trying to cut down on foreign trips. So at the moment, I'll be going to Germany in June. Aside from that, I'll be going to France in May. I think that's all I can recall at the moment.

Q: What's your trip to France for?

A: I'll be teaching in an advanced vaccinology course in Annecy.

Q: Where?

A: Annecy. What's that? I'm sorry. A-N-N-E-C-Y. It's a town in France.

Q: Who is sponsoring this course?

A: Well, it's sponsored by the University of Geneva and the Gates Foundation.

Q: Anybody else?

A: No. Basically those are the funders.

Q: And your trip to Germany, what's that for, Doctor?

A: I'll be going to visit a biotechnology company that is trying to develop vaccines based on RNA.

Q: Do you have a position or affiliation with that company?

A: I'm simply on their scientific Board.

Q: One? And your trip to India, purpose of that

A: To discuss vaccination against chikungunya, a virus which is epidemic in India and in South America.

Q: And who are those discussions with?

A: Well, it's under the aegis of an organization called CEPI, which is a coalition to develop vaccines against epidemic diseases. So it's an organization that's received funding from various governments to meet the challenges of epidemic diseases like Ebola and chikungunya, et cetera.

Q: This trip also include meeting with vaccine developers?

A: Well, they will be present at the meeting. They will come and present the results of their efforts to develop a vaccine against chikungunya.

Q: Any trips planned in the United States for 2018?

A: Wish I had known to bring my calendar. I have no trips planned this month or actually next month. But I will be going to some NIH-sponsored meetings in March, as I recall, and there's a vaccine conference in Washington in April that I'll be going to.

MS. NIEUSMA: When you say "Washington," do you mean Washington state or District of Columbia?

THE WITNESS: District of Columbia. In May I'll be going back to France for the advanced vaccinology course. That's as much as I can remember at the moment.

BY MR. SIRI:

Q: Okay. There might be others; you just don't have your calendar here today, right?

A: Right.

Q: And the NIH meetings, where are those taking place?

A: In Bethesda.

Q: How far is that from here?

A: From here?

Q: Yeah. Do you drive there?

A: Oh, no. I take the train to Washington and then the Metro to Bethesda.

Q: How long does that trip take?

A: The train is an hour and a half. Metro is maybe 20 minutes.

Q: What's the name of the plaintiff in this case?

A: Well, from what was said before, the plaintiff, I think, is someone named Schmitt. I've not followed -- as I've said before, I have not been involved in the legal details. So I don't know the names except from what I've heard.

Q: What's the name of the defendant in this case?

A: As I understand it, they're a married couple, but that's all I can tell you. So I presume they're both named Schmitt.

Q: What's the name of their child?

A: I do not know.

Q: How old is their child?

A: I do not know.

Q: Do you know whether the child has received any vaccines?

A: I do not know.

Q: The name of the child is Faith. I'll refer to the child as Faith during this deposition, okay?

A: Mm-hmm.

Q: Faith's father believes that Faith's mother was wrong to not have given Faith all CDC-recommended vaccines on time. Do you agree with the father?

A: Yes.

Q: Is it your understanding that the father wants Faith to receive all vaccines she has missed and continue to receive all CDC-recommended vaccines?

A: That is my understanding, yes.

Q: Do you agree with the father that Faith should receive these vaccines?

A: Absent any contraindication, yes.

Q: Sitting here today, do you know whether Faith has any contraindications?

A: I do not know.

Q: So sitting here today, you don't know whether Faith should or should not actually get these vaccines?

A: In the absence of a contraindication, Faith should receive the vaccines.

Q: But you don't know whether she has a contraindication?

A: I do not know the medical history of the child.

Q: What vaccines has Faith missed according to the CDC schedule that you believe she should get?

A: Well, the CDC's schedule includes the diphtheria, tetanus, pertussis, hepatitis B, haemophilus influenzae, polio, measles, mumps, rubella. I don't know how old she is, so I don't know, you know, where to stop. But there are vaccines recommended in preadolescents. So she should receive those when she reaches the appropriate age.

Q: So just so I got -- just to make sure I understand, you believe she should get the hepatitis B vaccine?

A: Yes.

Q: Rotavirus?

A: Yes.

Q: DTaP?

A: Yes.

Q: Hib?

A: Yes.

Q: PCV13?

A: Yes.

Q: IPV?

A: Yes.

Q: The flu shot annually?

A: Yes.

Q: IIV, we'll call it the flu shot?

A: At the moment, yes.

Q: I'm sorry. At the moment?

A: At the moment.

Q: What do you mean?

A: I mean that there are two influenza vaccines, one of which is recommended for this year; the other is not recommended at the moment but may be in the future.

Q: You think she should get the recommended one?

A: Yes.

Q: And you think she should get the MMR, I believe you said?

A: Yes. And varicella.

Q: And hepatitis A vaccine?

A: I'm sorry.

Q: And hep A vaccine?

A: And the hep A vaccine, yes.

Q: How many doses of hep B as a child do you recommend they receive?

A: Three.

Q: How many doses of rotavirus do you recommend?

A: Two or three.

Q: And you recommend Faith receive those, right?

A: Yes.

Q: And you recommend that she receive the three doses of hep B?

A: Yes.

Q: And how many doses of DTaP do you recommend she receive?
A: Well, currently at least three, then a booster and eventually another booster.
Q: How many doses of Hib do you recommend she receive?
A: Well, three are usually sufficient.
Q: How many doses of PCV13?
A: Three.
Q: And how many doses of IPV or an inactivated polio vaccine?
A: Three.
Q: How many doses of the flu shot?
A: Well, one per year.
Q: And how many doses of MMR?
A: At least two, yes.
Q: How many doses of varicella?
A: Two.
Q: And hep A?
A: Two or three. Two is often sufficient.
Q: And those are the doses that you recommend that Faith receive, correct?
A: Yes.
Q: For each of those vaccines we just went through?
A: Yes. And then there are the adolescent vaccines as well.
Q: And what are those?
A: Well, meningococcus is often recommended and also human papillomavirus vaccine to, especially if she is a girl, but it's also recommended for boys as well.
Q: And you recommend that Faith receive those as well as meningococcus and HPV vaccine?
A: Yes.
Q: Any others?
A: Well, I could look up the vaccine schedule, if you wish me to, but I am sure that I agree with all of the CDC recommendations.
Q: How about when she becomes an adult; would you recommend that she get all of the adult vaccines that are recommended by the CDC for adults?
A: Certainly, yes.
Q: What are the, can you please tell me the brand name and manufacturer for each of the hep B vaccines?
A: I do not try to memorize brand names. As I recall, Engerix is the most commonly used hepatitis B vaccine, which is manufactured by GlaxoSmithKline. There's also a vaccine manufactured by Merck. I don't remember the trade name at the moment. As I said, I don't try to memorize trade names.
Q: So for the hepatitis B, there's a vaccine manufactured by GlaxoSmithKline. Can we refer to that either as Glaxo or GSK today?
A: Mm-hmm. Yes.
Q: And there's one manufactured by Merck?
A: Correct.
Q: Rotavirus, what are the brand names and companies that manufacture those?
A: Well, actually, one of the rotavirus vaccines I developed, so I do know that the trade name is called RotaTeq. And the other one is called Rotarix.
Q: Who manufactured those?

A: I'm sorry.

Q: Who sells those, manufactures those?

A: Merck manufactures RotaTeq, and GSK manufactures Rotarix.

Q: How about DTaP, who -- what are the brand names or manufacturers for DTaP?

A: Oh, boy. Sanofi Pasteur manufactures DTaP, and so does GSK. I do not remember the trade names.

Q: How about the hepatitis B vaccine; can you tell me what are the brand names for those products and the manufacturer?

A: For hepatitis B?

Q: For Hib. I'm sorry.

A: For Hib?

Q: I apologize. Did I say hep B? I meant Hib. Which stands for what, by the way, Dr. Plotkin?

A: Haemophilus influenzae type B.

Q: Thank you. So -.

A: Well, again, my recollection is that Sanofi and GSK, yes, both manufacture Hib.

Q: And -- okay. And what about PCV13; what is the name of the product and the manufacturer of that vaccine?

A: I don't remember the trade name, but Pfizer is the manufacturer.

Q: What about the flu shot?

A: Oh, well, there are multiple manufacturers.

Q: Yes, there are multiple manufacturers of the shot. Let's, in terms of flu shots -- strike that. We're going to come back to the flu shot. We'll make it simple. Well, let me ask you this, actually, about the flu shot: What flu shots, are there any flu shots recommended for children under one year of age?

A: No. Six months usually is the time, the age at which influenza vaccines are recommended for children.

Q: Do you know who manufactures flu shots recommended for children under one year -.manufacturers. There are probably ten different influenza vaccines, not all of which have been tested in children.

A: For children?

Q: Yeah.

A: I don't remember which of the So there are relatively few for children, all of them manufactured in a chick embryo. But anyway, I don't -- I'm sure that the major manufacturers like Sanofi and GSK certainly manufacture influenza vaccines. There's an Australian manufacturer, CSL.

Q: But, I mean just for -- I'm sorry, Dr. Plotkin. Just for, by age group, do you -- let me make this simpler. Do you know, do you have a recollection of which flu shots are recommended for which age groups?

A: You mean which manufacturers?

Q: Right.

A: I don't, don't recollect.

Q: In terms of the, in terms of the IPV, the inactivated polio vaccine, who manufactures, what is the product name manufacturer for that?

A: I don't remember the trade name, but Sanofi and GSK both make IPV.

Q: And the MMR vaccine, what is the product name and manufacturer for that one?

A: Merck is the manufacturer. GSK also makes one, but Merck is pretty much the American manufacturer for MMR.

Q: And for varicella, the product name and manufacturer?

A: Well, Merck, again, manufactures varicella vaccine, and GSK also does.

Q: And then for the hepatitis A vaccine, who is the, what are the product names and manufacturers?

A: Hepatitis A, GSK is the biggest manufacturer of hepatitis A.

Q: Is there any -- got it. Okay. And then... How about the meningococcal vaccine; what's the product name and manufacturer for that one?

A: Meningococcal vaccines are manufactured at the present time by Sanofi, by GSK, by Pfizer. Those are the three.

Q: And how about the HPV vaccine manufacturer, the product name and manufacturer, please?

A: Merck and GSK both manufacture HPV vaccines.

Q: So every vaccine that you believe Faith should receive is produced by either Merck, Sanofi, GSK, or Pfizer, correct?

A: Yeah. That's pretty much the case. In this country, at the present time, there are a limited number of vaccine manufacturers because vaccine manufacture is difficult and costly.

Q: Would it be correct to call these four companies the big four vaccine manufacturers?

A: Yes, that's correct. Johnson & Johnson is attempting to come into the field, but they are not yet one of the major manufacturers.

Q: Have you received any payments from Sanofi or any of its related or predecessor entities?

A: Yes. Certainly.

Q: In what years did you receive payments?

A: Oh, geez. Well, first of all, as you should know, in the 1990s I was medical and scientific director of Sanofi Pasteur, and so obviously I was paid by them. And since then I've been consulting for manufacturers, for biotechs, for governments, for nonprofits, and essentially for anyone interested in vaccine development. And so I have been remunerated by companies, not by nonprofits, obviously, and that is essentially what I do.

Q: Is there a year since 1990 that you've not received any kind of payment or remuneration from Sanofi?

A: Probably not, no.

Q: How much did you receive -- what would you say is approximate total amount of payments and remunerations you've received from Sanofi during your lifetime?

A: Oh, my God. I have no idea. I'm sure it's a sizable amount of money. But I, you'd have to ask my wife, who's essentially my accountant.

Q: Is your wife the person that would have the records to know that amount?

A: Yeah. She probably would.

Q: Okay. Would you say it's more or less than a hundred thousand dollars?

A: Oh, I'm sure it's more than that.

Q: 500,000? Would you say it's more or less than

A: it is. Probably, yes. Over the years, I imagine

Q: Would you say it's more or less than a million dollars?

A: Well, again, I'm not prepared to answer this question, but I'm sure it's a considerable amount of money. And over the years, it could well be more than a million.

Q: Do you believe it could be a few million?

A: You know, Counselor, I cannot give you a precise figure. It is a considerable amount of money. I do not doubt. But I could not give you a specific number because I've never looked at it.

Q: I'm going to make a request for the documents to understand precisely how much you've received from Sanofi over the years.

MS. NIEUSMA: I mean, you guys can do any discovery requests that you want. If he doesn't have it with him today, he can't produce it right now.

MR. SIRI: Your objection is noted, Counsel. Thank you .

BY MR. SIRI:

Q: Has any entity in which you directly or indirectly have a greater than 1 percent ownership interest received any payment from Sanofi or any of its related or predecessor entities?

A: Could you repeat that question.

Q: Sure. Does any entity -- do you understand what I mean by the term "entity," Dr. Plotkin?

A: Are you talking about me personally or -.

Q: When I say, I'm asking if you understand what the term "entity" means in that question.

A: No.

Q: Okay. Great. So when I use the term "entity," I mean it to include any business, sole proprietorship, company, LLC, LLP, limited liability company, organization, and so forth. Is that clear what "entity" means?

A: Yeah.

Q: So what I'm asking, has any entity, so any business company, that you've had directly or indirectly more than 1 percent ownership interest, okay, has any company like that received money from Sanofi?

A: Well, again, I'm not sure I understand the question. But I am the principal of a company called Vaxconsult -.

Q: Okay.

A: -- which essentially was organized to make things easier from the tax point of view. And that entity, if that's what you mean, has received payments from companies for whom I consult. So it's a device, if you will, to make things simpler for the accountant.

Q: Okay. So who owns Vaxconsult?

A: I do -- well, my wife and I do.

Q: And what percent do you own?

A: A hundred percent.

Q: Okay. And is there any other company -.and payments have been made to Vaxconsult by Sanofi?

A: Sure.

Q: And what's the total amount of payments that have been made to Vaxconsult by Sanofi?

A: Well, again, I do not have an exact number. I am sure that over the years, it's a considerable amount, but I cannot tell you exactly how much.

Q: Is there any other company in which you have an ownership interest that's received money from Sanofi?

A: No.

Q: You anticipate to continue to receive payments or any kind of other remuneration from Sanofi in the future?

A: As long as my health holds out, yes.

Q: What are those payments for?

A: For advice.

Q: Have you received any payments from Merck or any of its related or predecessor entities?

A: Yes.

Q: What year did you receive payments?

A: All I can say is since I stopped working for Sanofi, which was in early 2000s, I've consulted for essentially all of the major manufacturers. I do not know how much I received. But I have certainly received payments from Merck, from Glaxo, from Pfizer, and many other entities.

Q: So what was approximately the first year that you received payments from Merck?

A: Sometime in the 2000s.

Q: Would you say that you've received more than a hundred thousand dollars in payments/remuneration from Merck since then?

A: I have no idea.

Q: But you would have records that would be able to determine that amount, correct?

A: Yes. I doubt -- actually, I doubt that it's a hundred thousand, but I don't, I don't recall. As I said, my wife does the accounting, and I pay no attention to it.

Q: Do you anticipate receiving any payments or remuneration from Merck in the future?

A: Sure.

Q: You said that you received payments and other remuneration from GSK in the past?

A: Yes.

Q: When did those payments start?

A: Again, I cannot give you a precise year. But as I've tried to say repeatedly, since 2000, I've been consulting for many different entities, including GSK and the others.

Q: Do you expect to continue to receive payments or remuneration from GSK in the future?

A: Yes.

Q: I'll ask you the same question about Pfizer. You indicated that you have received payments or remuneration from Pfizer?

A: Yes.

Q: Do you remember when you first received any payments from them or any remuneration?

A: No, I don't recall what year that would be.

Q: And do you have a sense of approximately how much you've received?

A: No.

Q: Do you anticipate continuing to receive payments or remuneration from Pfizer?

A: Very likely.

Q: Now, all of the payments you've received from the big four vaccine manufacturers, as we've defined it, they were either made to you directly or through Vax -- I'm sorry. What was the -.

A: Vaxconsult.

Q: Or Vaxconsult?

A: Yes.

Q: Why don't we try this a little bit of a different way. Since it appears your memory of -.over longer periods of time is not as clear with regard to how much payment or remuneration you received from the big four, can you tell me, what is the total amount of payments in dollars you received in 2017, last year, from anyone or any entity involved in the development or sale of vaccines?

A: Of what?

Q: From any entity involved in the development or sale of vaccines.

A: Oh, my recollection is in the neighborhood of 200,000.

MR. SIRI: Sorry about that. My microphone wire got stuck. Let me just get this back on.

BY MR. SIRI:

Q: Do you own any stock in Sanofi?

A: No.

Q: Have you ever?

A: No.

Q: Do you own any stock options in Sanofi?

A: No.

Q: Have you ever?

A: No.

Q: How about from Merck, Glaxo, or Pfizer; do you own any stock in any of those companies?

A: No.

Q: Any stock options?

A: No.

Q: Has any educational or not-for-profit institution in which you have been involved received funding from Sanofi?

A: That's a very difficult question to answer. I don't inquire about the finances of the organizations that I work for or that I advise. So I find that question very difficult to answer. I imagine that some of them do, but I have no knowledge of the matter. Voices for Vaccines, for example, receives no funding from any of the pharmaceutical companies, and that is in order to avoid any suggestion of a conflict of interest. I think that's probably true for a number of the nonprofits I advise. But obviously it may not be true for companies.

Q: So you're saying Voices for Vaccines doesn't receive any funding from pharmaceutical companies?

A: None.

Q: What's your affiliation with that group?

A: Well, I was one of those who suggested that an organization of laypeople, as opposed to scientists, would be a good idea to oppose all of the nonsense that one sees on the web from anti-vaccination organizations.

Q: So it was your idea to create Voices for Vaccines?

A: It wasn't my sole idea. It was a suggestion that I made at a certain point. And it turned out that there were laypeople who were interested in promoting vaccines. Since then I've been on their advisory Board. But other than that, I have no role in the organization.

Q: But you were, from what I'm understanding, tell me if I'm correct, it sounds like you were a driving force in suggesting its creation and at least initially -.

A: Yes.

Q: -- getting it set up; is that correct?

A: Yes. Mm-hmm.

Q: I'm going to hand you what has been marked as Plaintiff's Exhibit 1.

(Exhibit Plaintiff-1 was marked for identification.)

MS. NIEUSMA: Amy, is that coming to my email?

MS. RUBY: It will be in just one moment.

MS. NIEUSMA: All right.

BY MR. SIRI:

Q: I'm going to hand you what's been marked as Plaintiff's Exhibit 1.

MS. RUBY: It's been sent. Hopefully it will come through.

MS. NIEUSMA: I'm sure it will. Got it.

MR. SIRI: Okay. Great.

BY MR. SIRI:

Q: Dr. Plotkin, do you recognize this as a printout from the Voices for Vaccines website?

A: Well, that's what it says. I don't read the website that often, but yes.

Q: Okay. And I see that it's got you listed on the scientific advisory Board -.

A: Yes.

Q: -- on the third page, correct?

A: Yes.

Q: Now, you see at the very end on the last page, Dr. Plotkin, see at the very bottom it says: Voices for Vaccines is an administrative product of the Task Force for Global Health?

A: Yes.

Q: And it receives funding from that organization, correct?

A: No. It does not receive funding. The task force was asked to do the -- what shall I say? -- the financial stuff required for an organization like Voices for Vaccines. But it does not contribute financially to Voices for Vaccines.

Q: Dr. Plotkin, I'm going to hand you what's been marked as Exhibit 2. This is a form 990 tax return for the Task Force for Global Health.

MR. SIRI: I'm not going to ask him questions until you've emailed it.

(Exhibit Plaintiff-2 was marked for identification.)

BY MR. SIRI:

Q: So I've handed you what has been marked as Plaintiff's Exhibit 2. It is the tax return for, the 990 tax return for the Task Force for Global Health. If you turn to the second page, do you see Section 4C?

A: Yes.

Q: Where there's expenses of $3,757,924?

A: Yes.

Q: Do you see that one of the groups receiving part of that funding was, in the last line, Voices for Vaccines?

A: I don't see where it says -.

Q: Last sentence in 4C.

A: Voices for Vaccines is expanding its educational outreach through new media and parenting networks, increasing its membership and its on-the-ground reach. So?

Q: If you go up to number four, Dr. Plotkin. Can you read what the items in that list are supposed to be describing?

A: Expenses, including grants, revenues. So?

Q: I'll read to it you, number four. It says, number four says: Describe the organization's programs, service, accomplishments for each of its three largest program services as measured by expenses.

A: Yeah.

Q: Are you claiming that this document does not represent that Voices for Vaccines received funding from the Task Force for Global Health?

A: As far as I am aware, that the Voices for Vaccines receives no funding from the task force. The task force under Dr. Alan Hinman has agreed to do the financial, whatever is required by the government to do the financial work, for Voices for Vaccines. But as far as I'm aware, it receives no funding from the task force or any other governmental or semi-governmental entity.

Q: So the task force does provide some support for Voices for Vaccines, correct?

A: It does.

MS. NIEUSMA: He already answered. He said he doesn't know.

MR. SIRI: Your objection is noted. Thank you .

BY MR. SIRI:

Q: The Task Force for Global Health, does the Task Force for Global Health receive funding from any of the big four pharmaceutical companies?

A: I do not know for a fact, but I doubt it. The task force, I know, secondhand. But I, I believe that they receive funding from CDC, but as far as I know, not from companies.

Q: Dr. Plotkin, I'm going hand you what's been marked as Plaintiff's Exhibit 3.

(Exhibit Plaintiff-3 was marked for identification.)

THE WITNESS: Yeah. So?

BY MR. SIRI:

Q: This is a -.

A: I see, yes, where it says: Funders. Well, I stand corrected. So the task force, then, does receive funding from companies. However, I don't see that has any bearing on its work for Voices for Vaccines.

MS. NIEUSMA: Where is that in the -- am I looking at the same exhibit you guys are?

MS. RUBY: You should have received Deposition Exhibit 3.

MS. NIEUSMA: It's a page from The Lancet?

MR. SIRI: No. Number 80. No. That's the wrong one.

MS. RUBY: Give me one second. Sorry.

MS. NIEUSMA: All right. (Brief pause.)

MR. SIRI: Counsel -.

MS. NIEUSMA: Yes.

MR. SIRI: What it is, it's a fact sheet printed out from the Task Force for Global Health, and on the left side it just shows the donors.

MS. NIEUSMA: Okay.

MR. SIRI: Dr. Plotkin's already, he's already -- I'm just going to ask him to read the donors and that's it. I assume -.

MS. NIEUSMA: All right .

BY MR. SIRI:

Q: So does this show that the Task Force for Global Health received funding from GSK?

A: Yes, it does. But I want to repeat that the Voices for Vaccines has studiously avoided receiving funding from any company. And the fact that the task force is doing its finances was only a matter of convenience and an offer from Dr. Hinman that they would do that because they have experience with filing tax returns, et cetera. And I do not believe, and I strongly do not believe that any of the funding to the task force passes to Voices for Vaccines.

Q: Does the Task Force for Global Health receive funding from Merck?

A: Yes.

Q: And from Pfizer?

A: Apparently, yes.

Q: So the Task Force of Global Health receives funding from pharmaceutical companies. And at the least, I'm understanding from you, provides some kind of administrative support services to the Voices for Vaccines, correct?

A: Correct.

Q: And one of the founding voices to create that organization was yourself, correct?

A: I was one of those who suggested it, yes.

Q: And you received remuneration from pharmaceutical companies, correct?

A: I do, yes.

Q: Does anybody that works for Voices for Vaccines -- strike that. Going back to what we were discussing, I had asked you earlier, has any educational or non-for-profit institution in which you have been involved received funding from Sanofi? And you indicated that would be difficult to answer. Can you tell me -- but you did indicate to me, and correct me if I'm saying -- I don't want to misspeak. But you indicated there are some groups that don't receive any funding from pharmaceutical companies, correct? And you mentioned -.

A: Correct.

Q: -- Voices for Vaccines as the main one?

A: Yes.

Q: Is there any other education or nonprofit institution in which you've been affiliated that you're aware of that does not and has not received funding from any of the, any vaccine company?

A: Well, I certainly advise the Gates Foundation. I advise the National Institutes of Health. I think those are the major institutions that are not in the business of, in the business of developing vaccines. And they do not receive funding from companies.

Q: Does the NIH hold any patents on any vaccine-related technology?

A: I believe they do, yes.

Q: Do they receive royalties from those patents?

A: I imagine they do, yes.

Q: To your knowledge, you're not aware of whether any of the other educational non-for-profit institutions outside of Voices for Vaccines, as you've said, Gates Foundation or NIH, that don't receive any money from any of the pharmaceutical companies?

A: I'm not sure I can answer that question categorically, but -.

Q: Just based on your knowledge. I mean, either you, you know, if you don't know, then...

A: I'm sure there are organizations that are not funded by industry. But whether -- I'm trying to think of ones that I've advised over the years. Well, the Seidman Foundation. I'm not sure whether they received funding from industry or not. But I don't normally inquire of the organizations that I advise where their funding comes from.

Q: Have you ever worked on developing a vaccine that was eventually used by the public?

A: Yes.

Q: Which ones?

A: Let's see. Well, rubella, rotavirus, rabies, and I made contributions here and there to anthrax, cytomegalovirus, varicella. That's all I can remember at the moment.

Q: The varicella vaccine, you're talking about VARIVAX?

A: Yeah.

Q: When you say you contributed to it, how did you contribute to development of varicella?

A: Essentially by showing how it could be used and demonstrating that it was safe and effective.

Q: Did you work directly with Merck on that?

A: I don't recall whether it was directly with Merck or not. Certainly it was the vaccine produced by Merck. But whether -- I don't recall that they actually funded my studies of varicella vaccine. But they were, they were the producers of the vaccine, certainly.

Q: Where were you working when you did this work?

A: At Children's Hospital of Philadelphia.

Q: Did Children's Hospital ever acquire any intellectual property rights on what was -.

A: For varicella, no.

Q: Have you developed or been part in any way in the development of any vaccine from which you have received any payment, revenue, or income related to the sale of that vaccine?

A: Yes. Although I should stipulate that all of the patents on vaccines that I've developed have been taken out by the institutions for which I was working and that they gave me -- and I stress that it was not a requirement, but they gave me part of the profits deriving from the patents.

Q: Which were those?

A: Sorry?

Q: Which vaccines are those?

A: Mainly rubella, rotavirus, and rabies.

Q: And the rubella vaccine that you developed is currently used as part of the MMR vaccine?

A: Correct.

Q: And this is one of the vaccines you believe Faith's pediatrician should purchase and administer to her?

A: Absolutely.

Q: What is the total amount of payments in any form you have directly or indirectly received from the sale of the rubella vaccine?

A: I cannot give you a figure. I would say that I do not doubt. But, again, I'd have to ask my wife. I do not doubt that they were substantial amounts of money, and similarly for rotavirus and rabies.

Q: Was it in the millions of dollars for rubella? Just rubella.

A: I don't think so. That's all I can say. I don't think so.

Q: Are you in the possession of documents that would illuminate how much you've received in payments from the sale of the rubella vaccine?

A: Probably. I hope they have been retained. I don't know. But I imagine.

Q: And do you continue to receive any payments from the sale or royalties or any other remuneration from the sale of the rubella vaccine?

A: Currently, I don't think so.

Q: When did it cease?

A: Oh, Jesus, I couldn't tell you exactly. Sometime during this century. I don't know. You know, if I had thought that this was going to be about my finances, I would have had my wife come along because I don't follow these things. And certainly what I've done has not been based on what remuneration I could receive from the work that I've done. So if you want financial details, I will have to collect them in some other form. But -.

Q: How do you think your wife would feel of you offering her up for a deposition?

A: I don't think she would like it very much.

Q: That wasn't a serious question.

MR. SIRI: Okay. I'll request those documents .

BY MR. SIRI:

Q: Now, do you have -- you said that you're not sure whether it was in the millions of dollars that you've received from the sale of rubella, correct?

A: Correct.

Q: But it could have been?

A: I doubt it, but it could have been. I don't think so.

Q: Who provided you those payments?

A: The Wistar Institute.

Q: Did it come from any other source other than Wistar?

A: I don't think so because the Wistar holds the patent.

Q: Were you listed as one of the patent -.

A: One of the inventors?

Q: One of the inventors?

A: I believe so, yes.

Q: But the Wistar was the assignee; is that right?

A: Yes.

Q: And so they received the -- they're the ones who had the, gave the license to Merck?

A: Yes. Yes.

Q: So Merck would pay Wistar, and then Wistar would remit some of that to you; is that correct?

A: That's correct. I'm trying to recall whether Children's Hospital was involved. I don't think so at that point because that was many years ago.

Q: And you indicated that you've also developed the rotavirus vaccine earlier. I believe you said it was RotaTeq?

A: Yes.

Q: That's, and I think you said earlier that's currently one of two rotavirus vaccines currently on the market in the U.S.?

A: Yes.

Q: And you obtained a patent for RotaTeq?

A: Wistar and Children's Hospital developed patents.

Q: Who is listed as the inventor or co-inventors?

A: Myself, Paul Offit and Fred Clark.

Q: Who are the assignees of the patent for RotaTeq?

A: Assignees, you mean who used the -.

Q: Well, you know, when you file a patent, there's usually an inventor listed and then there's who you, the patent is assigned to.

A: Well, the patents were taken out by Wistar and Children's Hospital, if that's what you mean.

Q: Okay. And so they were the ones who had the rights to the patent?

A: Yes.

Q: How much remuneration to date have you received from sales of RotaTeq?

A: I couldn't tell you exactly, but it's been a considerable amount.

Q: Has it been in the millions?

A: I hesitate to say exactly. It could be, but I really do not know.

Q: You were entitled -- so you indicated that Children's Hospital of Philadelphia, is that sometimes referred to as CHOP?

A: Yes.

Q: CHOP was entitled to receive revenue from the sale of RotaTeq?

A: Yes.

Q: What portion from the sale of RotaTeq was CHOP entitled to?

A: Well, as I understand it, 50 percent.

Q: And what percent of that 50 were you entitled to?

A: I don't know.

Q: Do you know how much revenue CHOP received from the sale of RotaTeq?

A: I do not.

Q: Did there ever come a time where CHOP sold its interest in the RotaTeq virus vaccine?

A: I believe so, yes.

Q: Do you remember how much approximately it was sold for?

A: No.

(Exhibit Plaintiff-4 was marked for identification.)identification.)

BY MR. SIRI:

Q: I'm going to hand you what is being marked as Plaintiff's Exhibit 4. This is a press release from Royalty Pharma. And the title of the press release is: Royalty Pharma acquires royalty interest in RotaTeq from the Children's Hospital Foundation for 182 million.

MS. RUBY: Ms. Nieusma, you should have that in just one second .

BY MR. SIRI:

Q: Looking at Exhibit No. 4, does that refresh your recollection of how much CHOP sold its interest in RotaTeq for in 2008?

A: Assuming it's correct, yes.

Q: Does that sound about right?

A: I have no idea, but presumably it's correct.

Q: Do you have any reason to doubt the authenticity of this press release?

A: No.

Q: Do you have any reason to doubt that CHOP sold its RotaTeq interest in 2008 for $182 million?

A: I have no reason to doubt it.

Q: Did you receive a portion of those proceeds?

A: I believe so, yes.

Q: What was that amount?

A: I could not tell you precisely. I really can't. I don't do these things for the money. And although it's gratifying to receive monetary awards, I don't personally keep track of it. Again, if I had realized this was going to be the tone of this deposition, I would have asked

my wife to come along .
BY MR. SIRI:
Q: You're here today opining that Faith should receive vaccines that are made by the big four pharmaceutical companies, correct?
A: I am, yes.
Q: Okay. And you didn't anticipate that your financial dealings with those companies would be relevant in that issue?
A: I guess, no, I did not perceive that that was relevant to my opinion as to whether a child should receive vaccines. Vaccines have to be made by somebody. And, of course, in this world they're made by pharmaceutical companies who make profits on vaccines. And the fact that they make profits on vaccines has no bearing on whether those vaccines are good for a child or not.
Q: So you think the fact that pharmaceutical companies make money on vaccines doesn't bias how they approach the promotion of their own products?
A: I imagine it biases them in favor of vaccines, but so does most of the scientific world.
Q: Are you saying most of scientific world is biased because of financial -.
A: No.
Q: -- conflicts of interest?
A: I'm saying most of the scientific world believes that vaccines protect children against serious diseases.
Q: Do you have a peer-reviewed study that actually supports what you just said?
A: Absolutely, yes.
Q: Okay. Good. We'll make a demand for that, too.
A: Well, you can certainly buy a copy of a Vaccines textbook, which contains thousands of references showing that vaccines work and are safe.
Q: So from the $182 million sale to CHOP -.that CHOP made to Royalty Pharma, do you believe that you received more or less than a million dollars?
A: I could have received more than a million dollars. I don't have an exact figure.
Q: You stated earlier your co-inventor on this was Paul Offit?
A: Yes.
Q: Were you entitled to similar remuneration as he was?
A: Yes.
Q: Are you aware that he has stated publicly how much he's received from that sale?
A: I am not aware that he has.
Q: If I told you he said that he received approximately $6 million, would that -.
A: Mm-hmm.
Q: -- would that help you recall how much you received?
A: Not really, but I believe whatever Paul has said I'm sure is correct.
Q: So is $6 million a lot of money, in your opinion?
A: Yes.
Q: If you received $6 million, do you think you'd remember?
A: Actually, Counselor, no. I hesitate to say this because it sounds as if I'm some sort of idiot. But I really do not follow what income I get. I have no doubt that it was a lot of money, but I cannot give you an exact figure. I actually do not read my own tax returns. I say that in complete honesty.
Q: How about the Wistar Institute; I believe you stated earlier they also were held to intellectual property on RotaTeq, correct?

A: Yes.

Q: Did there ever come a time -- and you receive a portion of the proceeds that Wistar receives, correct?

A: Yes.

Q: And you continue to receive payments from Wistar for the sale of RotaTeq?

A: I don't think I received anything in the last couple of years, but I have in the past.

Q: How much approximately have you received in the past?

A: I don't remember.

Q: Do you recall Wistar selling a portion of its royalty interest to RotaTeq?

A: I believe they have.

Q: Do you remember approximately how much?

A: No.

Q: I'm going hand you what's been marked as Plaintiff's Exhibit 5.

(Exhibit Plaintiff-5 was marked for identification.)

BY MR. SIRI:

Q: It's a PR Newswire article. Can you read the title, please?

A: "The Wistar Institute Sells Partial Royalty Interest in Merck's RotaTeq to the Paul Royalty Fund."

Q: Does that refresh your recollection of how much they sold their royalty interest?

A: No.

MS. RUBY: Ms. Nieusma, did you receive Exhibit 5?MS. NIEUSMA: I did. I believe Exhibit 5 I have, yep, just got it.

MS. RUBY: Thank you .

BY MR. SIRI:

Q: Can you please read the first sentence of the article, Dr. Plotkin.

A: The Wistar Institute today announced that it sold a portion of its anticipated worldwide royalty revenues from RotaTeq to an affiliate of the Paul Royalty Fund for $45 million.

Q: Does that refresh your recollection of how much they received for selling a portion of their interest in RotaTeq?

A: I know that they sold it. I don't have in my head how much they sold it for. But I presume this is correct.

Q: The Wistar Institute is entitled to what percentage of the sales from the RotaTeq?

A: I do not know.

Q: From this $45 million sale, any recollection at all of how much you received?

A: No recollection. I'm sure I received some.

Q: Do you think it was sizable?

A: I think it was probably sizable, yes.

Q: More than a few hundred thousand?

A: I think so. I don't have a figure in my head.

Q: Do you have documents that would indicate how much you received?

A: I would imagine so, yes.

MR. SIRI: We'll make a request for those as well .

BY MR. SIRI:

Q: Are you familiar with the Immunization Action Coalition?

A: Yes.

Q: What is your understanding of what this group does?

A: They promote vaccination through education and emails and meetings.

Q: Would you say it's one of the main advocacy groups for vaccines in this country?

A: I think it's an important one, yes.

Q: Does it receive funding from pharmaceutical companies?

A: I believe -- I think so. I'm not certain. I don't know exactly where their financing comes from, but I think they very well may.

(Exhibit Plaintiff-6 was marked for identification.)

BY MR. SIRI:

Q: I'm going to hand you what's been marked as Plaintiff's Exhibit 6. It's a printout from the Immunization Action Coalition web page showing their funding for 2017. If you could kindly take a look at that and the section that says, that lists the pharma company donors.

A: Mm-hmm.

Q: Are any of the companies listed there vaccine manufacturers trying to develop vaccines?

A: Yes.

Q: Which ones?

A: AstraZeneca, Glaxo, Merck, Pfizer, Sanofi, Seqirus.

Q: So all of them?

A: Yes.

MS. RUBY: Ms. Nieusma, can you confirm you received Exhibit 6.

MS. NIEUSMA: Haven't gotten it yet, but I should have it in just a second. Got it.

MS. RUBY: Thank you .

BY MR. SIRI:

Q: Do you know approximately what percent of Immunization Action Coalition's funding comes from those pharmaceutical companies?

A: No idea.

Q: Can you name me a major medical group, such as the American Academy of Pediatrics or similar, that you know does not receive any funding from any pharmaceutical company?

A: Well, inasmuch I do not know what organizations receive what funding, I really can't answer that question.

Q: Sitting here today, you don't know of one?

A: I don't know what funding, for example, AAP receives from manufacturers, no.

Q: So sitting here today, you're not aware of any medical group that does not receive any support from pharmaceutical companies, correct?

A: I am not aware of the funding of medical organizations and whether or not they receive funding from pharmaceutical companies.

Q: So just to recap, I think it would be correct to say that you've received in total from the companies that develop or manufacture vaccines payments or remuneration at least in the amount of a few million dollars, correct?

A: I think it's correct to say that since I left Children's Hospital in the 1990s, I have received considerable funding for my work in developing vaccines and in advising companies how to develop vaccines, and I have also given advice freely to organizations that could not pay me because I believe that vaccines are important to the health of children and adults.

Q: So the answer is yes?

A: The answer is yes, but I wish to say very clearly that none of the things that I have done have been done with the objective of gaining money. It has been my fortune that I have been rewarded financially for the work that I've done. But none of the things that I've done have been done for financial gain. And I resent very much the line of questioning that suggests that what I believe and what I've done have been done for financial reasons.

Q: Nobody is suggesting that, Dr. Plotkin. I'm just asking you -.

A: Baloney, you are suggesting that. That's -.

Q: You're suggesting that. Dr. Plotkin, you indicated that a lot of the remuneration you received is from the 1990s. Have you received any funding from the big four pharma companies or their predecessors before 1990?

A: I would say probably not. You know, it's very hard to remember that far back. But certainly not any substantial funding. I may have received honoraria for attending meetings in those days, but certainly nothing, nothing considerable. At that point I was working at the University of Pennsylvania and the Children's Hospital and the Wistar Institute and was, of course, paid by those entities.

MR. SIRI: Could you read the last answer back for me, please. - - . (Whereupon, the Reporter read back a preceding portion of the testimony as directed: "A. I would say probably not. You know, it's very hard to remember that far back. But certainly not any substantial funding. I may have received honoraria for attending meetings in those days, but certainly nothing, nothing considerable. At that point I was working at the University of PennsylvaniA and the Children's Hospital and the Wistar Institute and was, of course, paid by those entities.")

BY MR. SIRI:

Q: Did you receive any funding from any pharmaceutical company related to the development of vaccines before 1990?

A: I don't recall receiving any funding for the development of rubella vaccine before it was licensed and then funding passed through Wistar. As far as rotavirus is concerned, I did have grants, not personal money, but grants for rotavirus development from Sanofi. And I had no funding for rabies. That's as much as I can recall.

Q: But you indicated that you didn't get funding for the work on the rubella vaccine, right?

A: I don't believe I had any funding until it was eventually licensed by Merck.

Q: When was that?

A: That was about 1970 -- early '70s.

Q: So from the early '70s, you were receiving funding, you're saying, from Merck related to rubella?

A: No. Wistar was receiving funding.

Q: Wistar from Merck?

A: Yes.

Q: Got it. But before that?

A: Merck did not fund the development of rubella vaccine until it was licensed.

MS. RUBY: Ms. Nieusma, you should have Exhibit 7.

(Exhibit Plaintiff-7 was marked for identification.)

BY MR. SIRI:

Q: I'm going hand you, Dr. Plotkin, what's been marked as Plaintiff's Exhibit 7.

MS. NIEUSMA: Just got it .

BY MR. SIRI:

Q: Can you read the title of the article, please.

A: Attenuation of RA 27/3 Rubella Virus in WI-38 Human Diploid Cells.

Q: Who is the first listed author?

A: I am.

Q: What is the year of this publication?

A: 1969.

Q: And if you go to the, if you go to the summary -- you know what? Dr. Plotkin, let me -.may I -.

A: Oh, yes.

Q: Does it say there that Mr. Plotkin is a recipient of an award from Smith, Kline -- is that a predecessor to GSK?

A: Yes, it is.

Q: Okay. -- and French, Inc., Philadelphia, for research on rubella vaccine, correct?

A: Yes. Unfortunately, that was not the vaccine that eventuated; in other words, the RA 27/3 was not the really the product of any GSK funding.

Q: Does that refresh your recollection now of maybe what was an earlier time that you received funding from pharmaceutical companies towards development related to a vaccine?

A: Yes. I -.

Q: Okay.

A: I did have some funding from GSK, but they had their own candidate rubella vaccine.

(Exhibit Plaintiff-8 was marked for identification.)

BY MR. SIRI:

Q: Dr. Plotkin, I'm going to hand you what has been marked as Plaintiff's Exhibit 8.

MS. RUBY: Ms. Nieusma, did you receive that Exhibit 8?

MS. NIEUSMA: I'm sure I will.

MS. RUBY: It might take a second. It's Dr. Plotkin's Curriculum Vitae.

MS. NIEUSMA: I've got a copy of that already.

MS. RUBY: Thank you .

BY MR. SIRI:

Q: This is your CV, correct, Dr. Plotkin?

A: Yes.

Q: Did you update this CV recently?

A: I think it was updated last year, but I'm not sure exactly. It probably doesn't have every last publication.

Q: On the first page in the top right corner, do you see the date?

A: June 2017.

Q: Is that when it was last updated?

A: Yes.

Q: If you go to the end, I saw that you went, there are some articles here that were published in 2017 in which you're an author?
A: Yes.
Q: I think I count one, two, three, four, five, six, seven articles, correct?
A: I guess.
Q: Some of these were published within the last few months?
A: Mm-hmm.
Q: I think some of them were published in December or November, correct?
A: Yes.
Q: So this has been updated very recently, correct?
A: Well, June 2017.
Q: The articles, if you go to article 794, Rodrigues, Pinto.
A: Yeah.
Q: Do you know what month of the year that was published?
A: No.
Q: If I told you it was published after June, would that -.it.
A: Well, I guess my secretary must have added CV?
Q: When is the last time you reviewed this
A: Q Probably in June 2017.You provided this CV to the attorney for the defendant in this case?
A: Yes.
Q: It's quite a hefty CV, Dr. Plotkin. It's over 200 pages. I see there's 794 articles in it which you were the author, correct?
A: Yes.
Q: That's a lot of articles. I see a lot of honors, including Who's Who in America since 1978.
A: Mm-hmm.
Q: You have a number of faculty appointments at a number of universities I see here; one, two, three, four, five, six, seven, eight, nine, ten, 11, 12, 13. Any of the faculty appointments missing from this list?
A: I don't think so.
Q: I also see that there's, there's, you have a professor emeritus position at University of Pennsylvania and Wistar. Do you teach any courses there?
A: Yes.
Q: Do you continue to teach any courses?
A: Yes.
Q: What do you teach there?
A: Participate in the vaccine course at the university and essentially give advice to Wistar.
Q: And for the university, did you teach a course last semester?
A: Yes.
Q: Have you been doing that every year for the last -.
A: Pretty much, yes.
Q: -- few years? What's the name of the course?
A: Vaccines. I don't remember the exact name. But it's essentially a course in vaccines.
Q: How many days a week does the class meet?
A: Oh, two days. Two days a week.
Q: I see you have a number of hospital and administrative appointments. One, two, three

-- you have six of them, right? It looks like they're all at the Children's Hospital of Philadelphia and then Department of Pediatric -- any of your hospital administrative appointments missing from this list, Dr. Plotkin?

A: No, I don't think so. I do have an appointment at Johns Hopkins, but, yeah.

Q: What is that?

A: I'm an adjunct professor.

Q: Since when?

A: I think sometime in the 2000s.

Q: I see you have positions in industry listed, correct?

A: Yes.

Q: I see two of them. I see one is from 1991 to 1997, the medical and scientific director at
the Sanofi -.

A: Yes.

Q: -- right? And 1997-2009, executive advisor to the CO of Sanofi, correct?

A: Correct.

Q: But as discussed earlier, since 2009 you've also worked for Sanofi, correct?

A: I have, yes.

Q: And you worked for Merck?

A: Yes.

Q: And Glaxo?

A: Yes.

Q: And Pfizer?

A: Yes.

Q: How come those aren't listed here, Dr. Plotkin?

A: Well, they are consultancies. They're not official appointments. I don't have a, let's say, a
title at Merck. I'm simply a consultant to them. So it's not in my CV.

Q: So in providing this CV to your, to defendant's counsel, you didn't think disclosing
your affiliations with the very companies whose product you're saying Faith should receive, her pediatrician purchase and provide to her, was necessary to disclose?

A: The CV -.

Q: Strike the question. Let me ask you this: Are you willing to update your CV to disclose
all of the connections you have with the big four pharmaceutical companies?

A: Yes, of course. The CV is -.

Q: Okay.

A: -- created for, not for the, for legal purposes. This is created to inform people who want
to know about my papers and my appointments at various universities.

Q: You provided this to defendant's counsel, correct?

A: Yes.

Q: To show your experience as relevant to being an expert witness in this case, correct?

A: To show my experience as in the field of vaccines, yes.

Q: What is Dynavax Technologies?

A: Dynavax is a company that is working on adjuvantation of vaccines and has recently
licensed a hepatitis B vaccine that is more immunogenic than the current vaccines.

Q: This is a for-profit company?

A: Yes.

Q: Right. And it's involved in the development of vaccines, right?

A: Yes.

Q: You're on the Board of directors of this company, correct?
A: Correct.
Q: That affiliation is not disclosed on the CV, correct?
A: It's not on the CV, no.
Q: What is VBI Vaccines?
A: Variation Bio.
Q: Okay. And what is that?
A: That's a biotech developing vaccines.
Q: And this is a for-profit company as well, correct?
A: Yes.
Q: And you are also on the Board of Directors of this company, right?
A: Yes.
Q: And that affiliation is not disclosed in your CV, correct?
A: It is not in my CV, no.
Q: What is MyMetics?
A: MyMetics is a biotech in Europe. Actually, I haven't done anything for them in at least a year now. But I think I'm still officially on their Board.
Q: You're chairman of their scientific advisory Board, correct?
A: As I said, I haven't done anything for them for at least a year. So if that is correct, that's sort of an old thing.
Q: But they're a for-profit company?
A: Yes.
Q: And how long were you on their Board?
A: Couple of years. I don't remember exactly.
Q: But that affiliation is not on your CV, correct?
A: No.
Q: Dynavax Technologies, what have you done for them?
A: Dynavax, I've been on their Board.
Q: You attend the Board meetings?
A: Not recently, but, yes, in the past.
Q: Have you advocated on their behalf?
A: Yes.
Q: Have you done that in any government meetings, for example?
A: Yes. Yes.
Q: To seek licensure of the vaccine?
A: Yes. It was just licensed.
Q: And so you were advocating as a Board member of a technology company to get licensure of a new vaccine, correct?
A: Yes.
VIDEO OPERATOR: We have five minutes left on the disc.
MR. SIRI: Okay.
BY MR. SIRI:
Q: Inovio Biomedical Corp., what's that?
A: That's a biotech that's developing vaccines based on DNA.
Q: And is this a for-profit company?
A: Yes.
Q: And what is your affiliation with the company?

A: I'm on their Board.

Q: And was that affiliation disclosed in your CV?

A: No.

Q: What's CureVac AG?

A: It's also a biotech.

Q: Is it a for-profit company?

A: Yes.

Q: Is it involved in the development of vaccines?

A: Yes.

Q: What's your affiliation with that company?

A: I'm on their Board.

Q: Did you, is that affiliation disclosed in your CV?

A: No.

Q: What is Syn, S-Y-N, Vaccine?

A: Actually, I'm not sure about that, about that name. But as I recall, it's a company trying to develop synthetic vaccines.

Q: What's your affiliation with that company?

A: Actually, I don't recall that -- I've certainly helped them, but I don't recall that I have a Board position or whether I'm officially on the Board or not. I haven't had contact with them for some time.

Q: What is GeoVax Labs?

A: It's also a biotech.

Q: Is it a for-profit company?

A: Yes.

Q: Is it involved in the development of vaccines?

A: Yes.

Q: What's your affiliation with that company?

A: I've been an advisor, and I think I'm officially on their Board. They're trying to develop a vaccine against HIV.

Q: Was this association disclosed in your CV -- no, right?

A: No. I don't have my consultancies on my CV.

Q: You're on the Board of these companies, correct?

A: Yes.

Q: What is GlycoVaxyn AG? That's G-L-Y-C-O, then capital V, A-X-Y-N AG?

A: It was a biotech in Europe.

Q: Is it a for-profit company?

A: It was.

Q: Okay. Was it involved in the development of vaccines?

A: Yes.

Q: well? Were you on the Board of this company as

A: Yes.

Q: Did you, is that disclosed in your CV?

A: No.

Q: What is Adjuvance Technologies? That's A-D-J-U-V-A-N-C-E, Technologies?

A: It's a company trying to developed adjuvants for vaccines.

Q: Is it a for-profit company?

A: Yes.

Q: You're on the Board of this company as well, right?

A: Yes.

Q: And that affiliation isn't disclosed in your CV either, right?

A: No.

Q: What is BioNet-Asia?

A: A company developing a new pertussis vaccine.

Q: This is a for-profit company as well?

A: Yes.

Q: And you're on the Board of this company as well?

A: Yes.

Q: That affiliation also wasn't disclosed in your CV, correct?

A: Correct.

Q: What's Abcombi -- that's A-B-C-O-M-B-I -.Biosciences?

A: I haven't heard from them in a long time. Actually, I'm not even sure -- I mean, I had an interview with the founder once. Whether he listed me as a Board member, I don't know. I haven't heard from him in a long time.

Q: It's a for-profit company?

A: I really have no idea. I assume it is, but I don't know.

Q: I should say that I'm spelling them out for the benefit of the court reporter. I assume you know the spelling. I'm just doing it for the benefit of the court reporter. What's Hook-ipa Biotech? That's -.

A: Oh, Hookipa?

Q: Thank you.

A: Yeah.

Q: H-O-O-K-I-P-I-A [sic] Biotech.

A: Yes. It's a European biotech.

Q: Is it a for-profit company?

A: Yes.

Q: And it's involved in the development of vaccines?

A: Yes, hopefully.

Q: And you're also on the Board of this company?

A: Yes.

Q: And that affiliation also wasn't disclosed in your CV, right?

A: No.

Q: You mentioned one of the companies was in the process of developing a new, trying to develop a new pertussis vaccine. Which company was that?

A: BioNet.

Q: Thank you. Why are they trying to develop a new pertussis vaccine?

A: Because the problem with current acellular vaccines is that, although they are protective, the protection doesn't last as long as we would like. And BioNet has developed a component of pertussis vaccine that should give longer-lasting responses.

Q: How long does the current immunity last from the current acellular pertussis vaccine?

A: Well, it lasts for probably on the order of five years, but the efficacy diminishes after two years or so. And the result is that there have been more pertussis in adolescents than we would like.

Q: So when you say after five years immunity is gone in two years, the efficacy, do you mean after -- how many dose -- the four- or five-dose DTaP series?

A: Well, I should go into some detail. The first -.
VIDEO OPERATOR: Thirty seconds .
BY MR. SIRI:
Q: Well -.
A: The first three doses are given -.
Q: You know what? I apologize. The, it's about the run out, and I don't want to give the videographer a hard time.
VIDEO OPERATOR: This ends disc one of the deposition of Dr. Stanley Plotkin. We're going off the record. The time is 10:32.

(Brief recess.)

Part 2

VIDEO OPERATOR: This is the beginning of tape No. 2 of the deposition of Dr. Stanley Plotkin. We are on the record. The time is 10:42.
MR. SIRI: Thank you .
BY MR. SIRI:
Q: Apologies, again, for cutting off the answer to your last question. The tape needed to be changed.
MR. SIRI: If you could kindly read back the last question to give Dr. Plotkin an opportunity to respond. - - . (Whereupon, the Reporter read back a preceding portion of the testimony as directed: "Q. So when you say after five years immunity is gone in two years, the efficacy, do you mean after -- the four- or five-dose DTaP series? "A I should go into some detail. The first -. "Q Well -. "A The first three doses are Stanley Plotkin, M.D. given -. "Q You know what? I apologize. It's about the run out.") THE WITNESS:
So pertussis vaccine is given in three doses in infancy and is quite protective during the childhood or infancy years. Then there's a booster dose given before school entry, and that results in protection, pretty good protection for two, three years, but then begins to fade when the child reaches eight or nine years. And a dose is recommended in preadolescents. And there in particular what's been found is that with the so-called acellular vaccines, that after two or three years, that the efficacy diminishes considerably. And so there are efforts to try to improve that persistence of efficacy. And BioNet is one of the companies that is, in effect, trying to develop a longer-lasting acellular pertussis vaccine. There are other companies also working to improve the vaccine for adolescents .
BY MR. SIRI:
Q: So the last vaccine recommended for adolescents is around what age, of DTaP or diphtheria-, tetanus-, and pertussis-containing vaccine?
A: Thirteen, 11.
Q: Eleven, 13?
A: Thirteen.
Q: And did I understand correctly that a few years after that last dose, the most folks who have gotten that vaccine are no longer immune to pertussis?
A: Well, "most folks" is perhaps a bit of an exaggeration -.
Q: Okay.
A: -- but it depends on the study. But certainly I would say that the high effectiveness that's seen initially after the vaccine diminishes considerably by five years.

Q: What do you mean by "considerably"?

A: Well, so it falls somewhere between 30 to 50 percent protection, so it's not nearly as good as after the vaccine dose is given.

Q: So after the last vaccine dose in adolescents, five years later only 30 to 50 percent of people are -- receiving these CDC-recommended childhood schedule are protected from pertussis?

A: Yes.

Q: How about ten years out?

A: I'm not sure there are many studies that go that far out. But I would imagine that the protection is diminished considerably by that time.

Q: So most adults aren't protected for pertussis?

A: Not unless they've received a booster dose. But that being said, it becomes complicated because if they are infected with the organism that causes pertussis, even if they are not ill because of it, they will get a natural booster, and so they may not have symptomatic pertussis. Pertussis is not uncommon in adults. But the epidemiology is not as well established as it is for children.

Q: But in terms of protection from vaccination from pertussis, most adults are not protected from the vaccination; you're saying they're, if they're protected, they're protected from exposure to the actual pertussis -.mind that pertussis as a disease is most important in the newborn and in children. And fortunately, we have very effective means of preventing pertussis in those highly susceptible individuals.

A: Yeah.

Q: -- is it bacteria?

A: Yes. But, you know, you have to bear in. Adults will have a cough disease, but they won't die of pertussis. So although we want to protect them as well, the main point of pertussis vaccine is to protect the newborn and the young child.

Q: So is it only really dangerous in the first, what, few months of life? Or -.

A: Yes. Infants with pertussis may frequently die of pertussis. And that's why immunization in pregnancy is now practiced. In other words, to provide passive immunity to the infant during the first months of life before the infant is vaccinated.

Q: And if the mother had been exposed to pertussis bacteria itself and had immunity that way, that would also confer immunity to the baby?

A: Yes. But one can't depend on that; whereas, if you give a dose of vaccine during pregnancy, you can depend on the antibodies passing to the infant.

Q: Does the cellular pertussis vaccine prevent the infection and transmission of pertussis in the person vaccinated with acellular pertussis vaccine?

A: Well, that's an area of active research. It appears that the acellular vaccines don't protect the individual from carrying the organism as much as the so-called whole-cell pertussis vaccines did. But those data are based largely on animal studies, and we don't really have a lot of human data to tell us whether the animal results are true in humans or not. But there is a concern that the acellular vaccines may not protect an individual from passing the organism to another individual even if the vaccinated person doesn't get sick himself or herself.

Q: What animals are used in those studies?

A: Baboons.

Q: Why were baboons used?

A: Why were baboons used? Because they are susceptible to pertussis, and obviously they are close to humans.

Q: Would those experiments be ethical to do with people as opposed to baboons?

A: Well, I'm not sure it would be ethical to infect someone with pertussis. That would require an ethical committee to consider what, how the experiment would be done. For example, if someone were infected with pertussis and then given antibiotics soon after administration of the organism, that could be ethical because the antibiotics would cure the individual before he or she becomes ill.

Q: Wouldn't that mess up the study, though?

A: Sorry?

Q: Wouldn't that, but then wouldn't that mess up the study in terms of -.

A: It would certainly influence the study. But it could allow us to determine whether an individual who has been vaccinated with the acellular vaccine can pass the organism, despite the vaccination, to another individual.

Q: Has that study been done?

A: No, that has not yet been done. Q In terms of the study that was done with baboons, that study -.

A: Yes.

Q: -- could that study be done with human -.do you think any IRB approval could ever be obtained to do that study with humans?

A: To allow an individual to develop symptomatic pertussis? I don't think that would be approved.

Q: Okay. What was, so in terms of the baboon studies that were done, that's about as, those are about as good as you're going to get for those studies because you can't do the human studies, correct?

A: Well -.

Q: In terms of evidence about the transmissibility and infection of pertussis from -.

A: Yes, but -.

Q: -- after acellular pertussis vaccination.

A: Yes. But I, I believe that workers are trying to determine whether vaccinated individuals are still colonized by the pertussis organism. If they are colonized, then they probably could transmit to others. I mean, there's a lot of work going on in this field, including developing an attenuated Bordetella pertussis which could be given to boost immunity and, in particular, to prevent carriage. So as I said, this is a very active area of investigation.

Q: What was Merck's total revenue from vaccine sales in 2016?

A: No idea.

Q: Do you think it was in the millions?

A: I imagine so. But I certainly have no knowledge.

Q: Do you think it was in the billions?

A: I don't, do not know.

Q: Do you know what the, do you know what the global sales of vaccines were, approximately, last year?

A: My vague recollection is something like 30 billion.

Q: Thirty billion. Do you know what percent approximately Merck's share of that was?

A: No.

Q: Sanofi's?

A: No.

Q: Glaxo?

A: No.

Q: Or Pfizer?

A: No.

Q: Do you -- combined what, do you have a sense of what those four represent in terms of that $30 billion in vaccine sales?

A: Probably. I would guess, but it's purely a guess, 20 billion.

Q: And the increase in the vaccine market has been due to the fact that new vaccines give higher profits, correct?

A: Correct.

Q: Are you familiar with the New England -.strike that. If I told you -- in terms of the $30 billion, and you said approximately -- what percent did you say approximately you thought was from the big four vaccine makers?

A: I said 20. I really don't have an accurate idea, but that's my guess.

Q: Twenty?

A: Billion.

Q: Oh, billion. You said what percent of that was related from the four, to the four big vaccine manufacturers?

A: What I said was that I thought the overall income was 30, but that the big four probably account for 20. But that's, those are purely guesses.

Q: Then let's do this. When you say it's a guess, how off do you think you might be?

A: If it's a guess, how do I know how off I am?

Q: How did you come up with the 20 billion?

A: Because I vaguely recall having seen a paper with those numbers. But my memory may be incorrect.

Q: Are you familiar with the New England Journal of Medicine?

A: Yes, of course.

Q: What does an editor for this journal do, does?

A: What does an editor for the journal do?

Q: Yeah.

A: I presume that he edits articles that are submitted to the journal.

Q: What does the editor in chief do?

A: Selects articles to be published.

Q: What is your opinion about this, the New England Journal of medicine?

A: It is an influential medical journal.

Q: I'm going to read you a quote from a Dr. Edmond J. Safra, professor at Harvard Medical School and former editor in chief at the New England Journal of Medicine. And I'm going to ask you a question about it. Okay?

A: Yes.

Q: So the quote says: Conflicts of interest and biases exist in virtually every field of medicine, particularly those that rely heavily on drugs or devices. It is no longer possible to believe much of the clinical research that is published or to rely on the judgment of trusted physicians or authoritative medical guidelines. I take no pleasure in this conclusion, which I reached slowly and reluctantly over my two decades as the editor of the New England Journal of Medicine. Are you familiar with that quote?

A: No.

Q: Okay. Let me read you a different quote, again, by Dr. Angell, in which she blames the issue that I just quoted, the issues with truths in medical publishing, on individuals that use legitimacy of academia to push pharmaceutical company agendas. Here's what she said about those individuals. She says, quote: They serve as consultants to the same companies whose products they evaluate, join corporate advisory boards and speakers bureaus, enter into patent and royalty arrangements, agree to be the listed authors of articles ghostwritten by interested companies, promote drugs and devices at company-sponsored symposia, and allow themselves be plied with expensive gifts and trips to luxurious settings. Many also have equity interest in sponsoring companies. Are you familiar with that quote?

A: Yes. I think I have read that, mm-hmm.

Q: You consulted for the big four vaccine manufacturers, correct?

A: Yes.

Q: You're in the corporate advisory Board of numerous vaccine developers, correct?

A: Yes.

Q: You've received royalties from the sale of one or more vaccines, correct?

A: Yes.

Q: Have you received -- you have received royalties from the sale of one or more vaccines, correct?

A: Yes.

Q: You are listed as an author on at least one or more papers where individuals authoring papers receive compensation from vaccine makers, correct?

A: Would you repeat that question.

Q: Sure. Have any of your co-authors on any of the papers that you've published received compensation from pharmaceutical companies?

A: Presumably, yes.

Q: And you've taken numerous trips over the last 30 years to various parts of the world?

A: Yes.

Q: I'm going read you a list of acronyms. And for the record, could you please state what you understand each to be. This way we can have commonality in terms of language. HHS?

A: Health and Human Services.

Q: these. Okay. CDC. I know these, I know that you know This is just so that when I use the term "CDC" later we have it defined.

A: Centers for Disease Control.

Q: Thank you. Thank you. Have you ever been involved with the CDC?

A: Yes, of course.

Q: What's been your involvement?

A: Well, actually, I was an epidemic intelligence service officer in the 1950s, and I have served on committees. I've attended numerous meetings at CDC. I've worked or, let's say, collaborated frequently with people from CDC. CDC is the world's most important epidemiology organization.

Q: FDA?

A: Yes. I've actually done consultation for FDA and interacted with people on FDA, yes.

Q: And it stands for the Food and Drug Administration?

A: Food and Drug Administration, yes.

Q: And the FDA is an agency within HHS, correct?

A: Yes.

Q: And CDC's also an agency within HHS?

A: Yes.

Q: Okay. NIH?

A: Yes, of course. National Institutes of Health.

Q: Right. And you've been involved with the NIH?

A: Yes.

Q: And how have you been involved?

A: Served on committees, worked with people at NIH, scientific collaborations.

Q: NIH is an agency within HHS as well, correct?

A: Yes.

Q: HRSA?

A: I'm not sure -.

Q: Health Resources Services Administration?

A: Okay.

Q: They're also an agency within HHS, correct?

A: Yes.

Q: Any involvement with HRSA?

A: I don't think so.

Q: ACIP?

A: Well, yes. The Advisory Committee for Immunization Practices. I have attended their meetings since 1960s, probably.

Q: Have you ever served on the Board at ACIP?

A: On ACIP itself? No.

Q: Okay.

A: No.

Q: Have you served on any Board related to ACIP?

A: To ACIP? I've worked, I have participated in working groups which they have organized on specific subjects.

Q: What working groups were those?

A: Let's see. Mumps. Let's see. What else? Mumps was the most recent one. I can't recall for the moment. But anyway, two or three working groups that they've organized from time to time. A yellow fever was one.

Q: Ever work on a working group for rotavirus?

A: Actually, no.

Q: And measles?

A: Measles? No.

Q: Not measles. I'm sorry. Rubella?

A: No, not for ACIP, no.

Q: A different government agency?

A: No.

Q: Actually, that was for WHO. For the rubella?

A: Yes.

Q: And for rotavirus, did you serve on a committee -.

A: No.

Q: -- for any other governmental entity? Strike that. That's okay. Oh, and WHO stands for?

A: World Health Organization.

Q: Thank you. I don't know if I'm going to pronounce this acronym correct. You can correct me if I don't. Is it VRBPAC? VRBPAC? VRBPAC? How is it normally pronounced?

A: "VRBPAC." Vaccines and Related Biologicals Advisory Committee.

Q: And that's V-R-B-P-A-C?

A: Yeah.

Q: Any involvement with that committee?

A: I have testified, but not, I have not served on the committee.

Q: What did you testify there for?

A: On the, at least the last time concerned the Dynavax vaccine.

Q: Oh, the, for the company you're on the Board for?

A: Yes.

Q: And this was to try to seek approval of that vaccine?

A: Yes.

Q: Which ended up getting approved?

A: Yes.

Q: The NVAC?

A: National Vaccine Advisory Committee. I've given talks to the committee.

Q: Okay. About what?

A: About vaccines.

Q: Fair enough. Anything in particular about vaccines or particular vaccines?

A: No. Actually, there was more or less general. It was not pushing any particular vaccine, but relation to the administration and the development of new vaccines.

Q: Ever give a presentation about the vaccine market?

A: About the vaccine market? No.

Q: And so all of the agencies and committees we just listed, CDC, FDA, NIH, HRSA, ACIP, VRBPAC, and NVAC, they're all under HHS?

A: I believe so, yes.

Q: And what's the, what about IOM; what does that stand for?

A: Institute of Medicine, now the National Academy of Medicine.

Q: Have you ever been involved with IOM?

A: Well, I'm a member of the National Academy. So yes.

Q: Since when have you been a member?

A: Oh, gosh. Ten years, but that's just a guess.

Q: What is the National Childhood Vaccine Injury Act of 1986?

A: Well, that's, in effect, it funds the organization that, shall I say, receives requests from individuals who believe that they've been injured by vaccines and remunerates them if they decide that, that there was a possibility that the vaccine did cause injury.

Q: So if somebody is injured by a vaccine, this law provides that they submit a claim to Health and Human Services?

A: Yes.

Q: And Health and Human Services then adjudicates -.

A: Yes.

Q: -- and those claims are filed in something called the Vaccine Injury Compensation Program, correct?

A: Yes.

Q: Administered in DC?

A: Yes.

Q: So, and the respondent in those cases is HHS, the secretary of HHS?

A: Yes.

Q: And the secretary of HHS in those cases is represented by the Department of Justice?

A: Yes.

Q: To defend against claims that the vaccines cause injury, right?

A: I would say that they determine whether there is a reasonable possibility that the vaccine caused injury. They, I would say, are relatively open and will give an award if there is a reasonable possibility. When this was first organized -.

Q: Do you have a study that supports what you just said or any type of -.

A: About what?

Q: That they are very, that they are open to giving awards? Do you have any governmental report or any authoritative source, any kind of governmental report or similar that supports the assertion you just made?

A: Well, I don't know. I'd have to look that up.

Q: Okay.

A: But the principle was enunciated years ago by the, particularly by the American Academy of Pediatrics. And their idea, which I now think was a good idea, was that rather than have an adversary situation, that they would set up an organization whereby if there was a reasonable possibility of injury, that they would offer remuneration, as opposed to the situation where lawsuits were being filed against companies and having an impact on whether the company was continuing -- would continue to make the vaccine. At a certain point there were relatively few companies making vaccines. And so this is an idea which over the years I have realized was a good idea, because it removed the -- how shall I say? -- the oppositional part of the story and made it possible for people who thought that they had been injured to be remunerated, whether or not that was biologically the case.

Q: So is it your testimony that the national, that the Vaccine Injury Compensation Program is not an adversarial system?

A: It's an adversarial system in that people have to have some reasonable information base to say that a child, let's say, has been injured. Whether it's because of a vaccine or whether it's a chance occurrence fortunately does not have to be adjudicated under this kind of system.

Q: That's only if it's a table injury, correct?

A: Yes.

Q: But if it's not a table injury, then the petitioner would need -.

A: Yes.

Q: -- to show that it was the vaccine that caused the injury?

A: Yes.

Q: So this is, I'm going to refer to this as the 1986 act. This is the act that gave vaccine manufacturers immunity from liability.

A: Yes.

Q: And you have to -- yeah, okay, for injuries caused by vaccines.

A: Mm-hmm. Yes.

Q: What is a bacteria?

A: It's a microorganism which has certain properties. It has a cell wall. And it has DNA within, within the organism. And it can, depending on what bacteria it is, it can multiply in humans and sometimes cause disease.

Q: How does it replicate?

A: It divides. It has mechanisms for dividing and multiplying.

Q: What is a virus?

A: A virus is a DNA or RNA molecule with properties to produce proteins and to replicate in cells and make more of it and is capable of causing disease under certain circumstances.

Q: When you say "replicate in cells" -.

A: Yes.

Q: -- do you mean in the host, the person that it infects?

A: Yes.

Q: So it takes over the person it infects own cellular DNA material?

A: Well, it doesn't take over the DNA necessarily, but it is able to replicate in cells that which, of course, have DNA. Not all viruses require that that they influence the DNA of the cell. But they all are able to replicate in the cytoplasm or in the nucleus of the cells of the host.

Q: And in that fashion, they will spread from cell to cell?

A: Yes.

Q: By duplicating themselves into more and more cells in the body?

A: Yes.

Q: And the virus DNA will, you said it can be either DNA or RNA?

A: Yes.

Q: And those DNA and RNA pieces, they provide coating for protein structures?

A: Yes.

Q: Those protein structures are typically, DNA creates protein structures that are important for regulating bodily functions?

A: Well, the virus is -.

Q: I mean DNA in general. I'm sorry.

A: Oh, DNA in general, yes. DNA in general codes for RNA, which then codes for proteins.

Q: Essential for human life?

A: Yes.

Q: And is DNA shared across humans, meaning is there similarity between the DNA sequence in different people?

A: There are similarities, yes, and there are differences.

Q: What percent of, you know, is the, similarity is there between human DNA amongst individuals?

A: Well, there are mostly similarities; but there are, of course, differences. That's why we are each different from one another.

Q: I've read -- tell me if this is not accurate -- that human DNA is approximately among individuals 99.9 similar among different people -.

A: Yeah.

Q: -- is that correct?

A: Yes.

Q: Okay.

A: But that still allows for differences.

Q: Right. Some of us have different eye color.

A: Mm-hmm.

Q: Yes?

A: Sorry. Yes.

Q: Do all humans and mammals -- strike that. What is the percentage of similarity between human DNA and the DNA in mammals of different kinds? Why don't we start with, why don't we start with -- sorry. Why don't we start with primates.

A: Well, the similarities are in the upper 90s, no doubt. But one has to appreciate that the differences that occur are critical and result in critical differences. So the fact that we're, let's say, 99 percent similar to chimpanzee doesn't mean that the differences are, the 1 percent difference is unimportant, because much of the DNA actually, the function of most of the DNA is unknown.

Q: So humans have approximately, between humans, have about 99.99 percent similarity in DNA and between humans and, I think you said, chimpanzees, about 99 percent similarity -.

A: Yeah.

Q: -- in terms of sequence?

A: Yes.

Q: What about for other mammals such as, let's say, between humans and chickens or cows or -.is there a similarity?

A: Well, there's similarity, certainly, but there are key differences. That's what I was referring to. Even though much of the DNA is the same, most of the DNA that we have, the function of which is unknown.

Q: And what percent would you say is similar?

A: With chickens, I don't know offhand.

Q: Cows?

A: Again, I don't know the number. But the point is that it doesn't require a large percentage

Q: Okay. Are you familiar with how the CDC of the DNA to be different.

A: Sure.

Q: What about guinea pigs?

A: (Indicating.)

Q: If you don't know, that's fine. just say you don't know.

A: I don't know.

Q: You can makes changes to its pediatric vaccine schedule?

A: Yes.

Q: Have you ever been part of that process?

A: Not part of the process, but certainly part of the discussion.

Q: In addition to changes to the CDC pediatric schedule voted upon by ACIP, correct?

A: Yes.

Q: What happens when ACIP votes for a pediatric vaccine to be added to the CDC's pediatric vaccine schedule for universal use?

A: It is adopted by various medical organizations and recommended to the physicians.

Q: And so the pediatricians around the country rely on those recommendations to decide whether or not to administer a vaccine?

A: Absolutely.

Q: What about children in the United States that can't afford the vaccines recommended by ACIP?

A: Well, until the present time, remains to be seen whether that will still be the case, the government pays for those children to receive vaccines.

Q: Is that called the Vaccines for Children Program?

A: Yes.

Q: And ACIP votes on whether or not to add a vaccine to that program, correct?

A: Yes.

Q: And when a vaccine is added to that program, the manufacturer is paid for the vaccine even if the child can't pay, correct?
A: Correct.
Q: Do you know what percentage of vaccines, pediatric vaccines administered in the United States are purchased from pharmaceutical companies using federal money through the Vaccines for Children Program?
A: Fifty to 60 percent.
Q: So when ACIP recommends a vaccine for universal use, it will essentially create a liability-free market of millions of children for the pharmaceutical company manufacturing that vaccine, right?
A: The act provides payment to the pharmaceutical company to manufacture the vaccine; that is correct.
Q: Are you talking about the 1986 act?
A: Yes.
Q: And they're not liable for injuries from the vaccines, right?
A: Unless it is the result of bad manufacture.
Q: But not for, if it wasn't, not for design defect claims?
A: Right.
Q: Meaning you can't sue a vaccine manufacturer claiming that they could have made the vaccine safer?
A: Correct.
Q: Who comprises the voting members of ACIP? Strike that. I didn't want the names. Let me ask it a different way. Are the individuals that serve on ACIP government employees?
A: No.
Q: Where do these individuals come from?
A: They come from all over the United States, and they are chosen because they have no conflict of interest; that is to say, they receive no funding from vaccine companies but are thought to know something about vaccines, nevertheless, with the exception of a community representative who is a layperson.
Q: So none of the members of ACIP have any conflict with regards to the manufacture, development, or -- of vaccination?
A: Right.
Q: When was the first rotavirus approved by ACIP for universal pediatric use?
A: That was, I don't remember the year, but my recollection is that was in the 1990s.
Q: If I tell you June 25, 1998, does that jog your memory?
A: Yeah, that could be right.
Q: On that date, June 25, 1998, you and your co-inventors, Paul Offit and Fred Clark, had already had a patent on the rotavirus vaccine, correct?
A: Yes.
Q: Were you at ACIP at the meeting that they first approved the first-ever rotavirus vaccine for universal pediatric use?
A: I believe I was.
Q: Was Fred Clark at that meeting?
A: I think he was. I'm not certain.
Q: Was Paul Offit at that meeting?
A: Yes.
Q: What was Paul Offit's role at that meeting?

A: His role? I don't remember whether he was still on the committee or not. I don't remember.

Q: He was on ACIP?

A: He was on ACIP, yes.

Q: He was a voting member of ACIP?

A: But I am confident that he was not allowed to vote on the licensure of RotaTeq or on the administration of RotaTeq.

Q: For the first, what was the first rotavirus vaccine that was approved for universal use in this country?

A: RotaTeq.

Q: Is that the rotavirus vaccine that you worked on?

A: Yes.

Q: There wasn't a rotavirus vaccine that was approved before that?

A: I don't believe so, no -- well, yes, there was a vaccine that had been developed at the National Institutes of Health that had been licensed, but was found to cause intussusception, and the manufacturer took it off the market.

Q: Paul Offit was on the committee and voted to approve that vaccine for universal use, correct?

A: Very likely, yes.

Q: At the time that he voted to approve that rotavirus vaccine for universal use, he was a patent holder with you and Fred Clark on a rotavirus vaccine, correct?

A: Yes.

Q: He didn't recuse himself from voting on recommending the rotavirus vaccine for universal use at that meeting, correct?

A: That's correct, which in a sense was voting against himself since obviously he was in favor of the vaccine that we were trying to develop. So in effect, he was voting for a competitor.

Q: When you have one vaccine for a given disease approved for universal use, wouldn't that make it easier to, then, have another vaccine for that same disease approved for universal use?

A: Assuming that the properties of the second vaccine were equal to or better than the first, yes.

Q: So approval of the first one paves the way for the second one, doesn't it?

A: It paves the way in the sense that if people believe that rotavirus disease is worth preventing, they will want more than one vaccine licensed so that in case there's a shortage of supply in one vaccine, there's an alternative.

Q: So there's, so there's, once you have one approved, it's a good idea to have a second one approved, then, isn't it?

A: It is, yes.

Q: Yeah. Are you aware of the many other conflicts of interest regarding the vote to approve the rotavirus vaccine for universal use that we've just been discussing that's been reported in a U.S. House of Representatives Committee on Government Reform report?

A: No.

Q: Are you aware that this report found that, quote, the overwhelming majority of members, both voting members and consultants, have substantial ties to the pharmaceutical industry, end quote? Well, I can't go back to 1998. But at the moment, my criticism of the ACIP committee is that many of the people on the committee do not have a very large knowledge about vaccines because they are eliminated from participating on the committee if they have any connections with, with industry. And I understand why that is the case, but it does result in the group of people who aren't necessarily the best informed. That being said, I agree with the idea that people who are on the ACIP should have no conflict of interest.

VIDEO OPERATOR: Watch your notes up against your microphone.

MS. NIEUSMA: Pardon?

MR. SIRI: The videographer was kindly advising me not to keep smacking my mic that's pinned to my tie.

MS. NIEUSMA: Got you .

BY MR. SIRI:

Q: Last question on this. Are you aware that the report, that this report by the U.S. House of Representatives' Committee on Government Reform concluded that ACIP, quote, Reflects, quote, a system where the government officials make crucial decisions affecting American children without the advice and consent of the governed?

A: I'm not aware of that report, and -.

Q: I'll give you a copy.

A: -- I do not agree with it.

(Exhibit Plaintiff-9 was marked for identification.)

BY MR. SIRI:

Q: I'm going to hand you what's being marked as Plaintiff's Exhibit 9. Happy to provide you a copy as well after the deposition that you can take home with you.

A: I will be interested in reading this. But I would say two things: One is that CDC certainly recently has leant over backwards to try to avoid people with conflicts of interest being on ACIP. And, second, that ACIP meets under public conditions; that is to say, the meeting is open to the public, the meeting is on the web, so that thousands of people, literally, can observe what goes on at the meeting and decide for themselves whether or not there's any hanky-panky. So although, as I said before, I might wish that people with more knowledge about vaccines be on the ACIP, by and large I think that they do a hell of a good job under public scrutiny.

Q: Are the working groups, are those also public?

A: They are not public in the sense that the public does not attend the working group. The working group does report back to the full ACIP, and the working group's presentations are presented publicly.

Q: But the discussions that the working groups have in conference calls leading up to ACIP meetings, those are not transcribed, are they?

A: They are not, no.

Q: Okay. And the members and individuals who participate in those working groups, right, which often lead to what ACIP then rubber-stamps, are permitted to have all forms and do have all forms of conflicts with industry, don't they?

A: They may. But I would contest the word "rubber-stamp." I've never seen the ACIP rubber-stamp a working group recommendation. Often it's just the opposite.

Q: You've also, you've also said that the meetings are available to the public. You've attended, you said, almost every ACIP meeting, correct?

A: Correct.

Q: Since, when was it, the '60s?

A: Yeah. Roughly, yes.

Q: And you attended the most recent one as well?

A: The most recent one being -- let's see. That would have been last October. Yes, I did.

Q: Were you presented anything at that meeting?

A: I presented the fact that I will no longer attend the meetings.

Q: Were you presented anything by the ACIP committee?

A: Yes.

Q: What were you presented?

A: I was presented -- well, I was told that there is a gavel with my name on it, that it will be used henceforth at the meetings.

Q: And they gave, so going forward, from this point forward, the gavel that's used at ACIP will have your name on it?

A: Correct.

Q: You gave a speech at that meeting, correct?

A: Yes.

Q: When they posted the video of that meeting on the Internet, did they include your speech, Dr. Plotkin?

A: I don't know, but I suppose they did.

Q: Well, you can check after this deposition on the website and see if your speech is there. I, we have not been able to find it.

A: Really? Wow. Too bad.

Q: Regularly at ACIP meetings, you get up and speak, correct?

A: I often do, yes.

Q: So you're given free, you're able to get up pretty much at any time and speak, aren't you?

A: Yes. Umm -.

Q: You don't have to wait for the public comment period, correct?

A: Correct.

Q: And that's also true of vaccine manufacturers; they also are permitted to get up and come to the mic and speak even not -- when there isn't public -.

A: Yes. They're often asked to answer questions that are being discussed.

Q: Isn't it true that they also get up and come to the front to speak even when not asked a question?

A: They may do so if they have, if it's a discussion about one of their products.

Q: But if members of the public want to speak, they have to wait until the public speaking period, correct?

A: Normally, yes.

Q: And when the videos are released, a lot of the conversations that occur between the pharmaceutical representatives and ACIP, do those also make it to the video that's released publicly?

A: As far as I know, the video contains all of the public hearings. In other words, if some-body comes to the mic, they are photographed; and as far as I know, they appear on the web. I must say that since I've been attending the meetings, I haven't really watched them; but I will in February when they meet again.

Q: So apart from the working groups that occur out of public sight, what other meetings or goings-about does ACIP engage in that's outside of the scrutiny of the public?

A: Aside from working groups, I'm not aware that they do have anything that's not public. I suppose they meet at lunchtime, and I don't attend those discussions. But that's all I know.

Q: Billions of dollars' worth of rotavirus vaccine have been sold to date, correct?

A: I believe so. I'm not acquainted with the sales figures.

Q: Does vaccination create a systemic change in the body?

A: Vaccination creates a change in the immune system of the body.

Q: Is that supposed to be system-wide, meaning if I get vaccinated in my arm but I'm infected in my toe, am I still supposed to still be immune?

A: Yes.

Q: So would you say, is it correct to say that vaccination is intended to create a systemic change in the body, throughout the body?

A: It's intended to create a systemic change in the immune system of the body.

Q: In the immune system everywhere in the body?

A: The immune system is expressed everywhere in the body. Yes. The immune system consists of antibody-producing cells and cells that are able to influence other cells.

Q: So the -- can you read back the last answer. - - .

(Whereupon, the Reporter read back a preceding portion of the testimony as directed: "A. The immune system is expressed everywhere in the body. Yes. The immune system consists of antibody-producing cells and cells that are able to influence other cells.")

BY MR. SIRI:

Q: Okay. Does the immune system comprise of more than antibody-producing cells?

A: It also has, also includes what are called T cells that are able to kill infected cells, for example, and to secrete substances that also have an effect on immunity.

Q: Is that referred to typically as cellular immunity?

A: Yes.

Q: And the immunity conferred by vaccines that you were talking about earlier is called -.

A: Humoral immunity, yes.

Q: Thank you. Appreciate that. Humoral immunity?

A: Yes.

Q: Okay. So humoral immunity creates antibodies, and it's called humoral because it originates from the bones? Is that kind of where the name derives from?

A: Well, the name derives from the ancient term "humors." But, in effect, it means antibodies that circulate throughout the body and can impact against infecting organisms.

Q: And the systemic change that you've described is supposed to last years, if not a lifetime -.

A: Yes.

Q: -- correct, from vaccination?

A: Yes.

Q: When you say "interact with other cells," when you say that the immunity created by vaccines creates antibodies which then interact with other cells, can you describe that a bit more? What do you mean by "interact with other cells"?

A: Well, the T cells, as I said, are able to attack infected cells in the body by a variety of mechanisms. They may actually directly kill those infected cells by direct action, as it were, or by secreting substances that can kill the cells. And they also influence cells to respond to the infection so that the infection doesn't continue to spread and impact on the individual's health.

Q: And how do the cells respond to the infection? Can you describe that?

A: You mean the patient's own cells?

Q: I thought that's what you were referring to in your explanation.

A: Yeah. The T -- the -- do you mean the infected cells or the T cells that are acting on the infected cells?

Q: Let's start with the T cells.

A: Well, the T cells, as I've said, have a variety of functions. They can secret substances that will kill an infected cell, or they can influence actually the antibody-producing system. They have impacts on a variety of ways in which the body protects itself against infection. There are cells called natural killer cells, for example, that can help protect an individual against an infection. And the T cells can influence the natural killer cells. So it's a complicated system by which the body responds to an infection or to a vaccine which allows the individual cells to be ready for an infection if it occurs.

Q: Modern immunology, though, doesn't fully understand that full cascade, correct?

A: I'm sorry.

Q: I said modern medicine, modern immunology, does not fully understand the complete sequence of events in terms of going from vaccination to immunity, correct?

A: Well, science never completely understands anything. But we know a great deal about how the body responds to vaccines or to infection, and that knowledge is growing every day. So, of course, we don't completely understand anything, including how the sun works. But that doesn't prevent us from using knowledge.

Q: What about its effects on other body systems? Can creating this immune response also have effects not only on creating antibodies to target cells that have been infected, but can it also have other bodily changes, other effects that are either known or unknown?

A: That's such a hypothetical question; I'm not sure how to answer it. Is an immunized individual any different than an unimmunized individual? Yes. Does the fact that the individual is immune have an effect on his or her general health? I'm not aware that that's the case. Remember that vaccines are, in effect, mimicking what happens after natural infections in many cases, but without causing the complete range of disease that the organism causes.

Q: So vaccines are just nothing more than a piece of the virus or bacteria; is that it? Is that all they contain?

A: Depends on the vaccine. The, that is to say, whether it's a live vaccine or a killed vaccine. The killed vaccines may only have small parts of the organism that they're protecting against. The live vaccines contain the whole organisms but altered so that they don't cause disease.

Q: Before vaccines are licensed, they go through clinical trials to confirm their safety, right?

A: Correct.

Q: These clinical trials assess if there are any harms caused by the vaccine, correct?

A: Yes.

Q: Was the DTP vaccine withdrawn from the U.S. market?

A: The whole-cell -.

Q: The DTP -.

A: -- pertussis vaccines have been withdrawn, yes.

Q: Because of safety concerns, right?

A: Because they cause significant fever and convulsions, febrile seizures. And they were, it was decided that it would be better to have a pertussis vaccine that didn't cause that type of reaction. So they were taken off the market, not because they were not working; quite the opposite, but because of safety concerns. Now, I do have to point out that aside from the U.S. and Europe, whole-cell pertussis vaccines are still used in the vast majority of countries in the world, and they are getting along just fine with those vaccines.

Q: Are you familiar with Peter Aaby, Dr. Peter Aaby?

A: Yes, of course.

Q: Didn't he recently publish a paper in which he looked at children who received DTP vaccine in the first six months of life versus children who received no vaccines in the first six months of life and found that those that received DTP died at a rate of ten times that of the unvaccinated?

A: I don't remember the exact figures. But you have to take into account that Peter Aaby -- I had many discussions with Peter Aaby. Peter Aaby's work is done in a, in non-placebo-controlled ways; that is, his studies are observational. Second point is that those studies have been examined more than once by World Health Organization committees. And their judgment has been that the effects of the pertussis vaccine in particular are not sufficiently documented to be acceptable or to change vaccination practice. So WHO does not recommend against the use of whole-cell pertussis vaccines; quite the opposite. They do recommend them.

Q: You said non-placebo-controlled. What do you mean?

A: I mean that essentially what Peter does -.and I'm not criticizing him because obviously it is very difficult to do, but he doesn't have randomly vaccinated or children who randomly receive pertussis vaccine or don't receive pertussis vaccine. What he has is, he follows children who have received this or that or the other vaccine and tries to draw conclusions from what he sees. But in the absence of random administration, you don't know for sure whether it's the vaccine or other factors that are operating.

Q: So in the study that I mentioned to you, if the children either were exposed to DTP and unexposed were randomized, that would make the study valid?

A: Yes. And, again, the WHO has at least twice gone over Peter's studies and has decided that they are not of sufficient proof to change their recommendations.

Q: Do you have a copy of those reports from the WHO?

A: Oh, gosh.

MR. SIRI: Because I'm going to make A demand for those WHO reports .

BY MR. SIRI:

Q: Do you remember when those reports came out?

A: Within recent years. I don't remember the year.

Q: More than a year ago?

A: Probably, yes.

Q: Peter Aaby's study just came out last year?

A: Well, I imagine WHO will reconsider them. But his studies suggesting that pertussis may, vaccine may increase mortality have been around for a while. It's not the first study that he's done. Also, one has to appreciate the context. By that I mean that he's also shown or attempted to show that live vaccines like measles vaccine has a very positive effect on mortality; in other words, that in his observations, those who received measles vaccine suffer from fewer diseases in general and have a lower mortality. And that effect has actually been confirmed immunologically. So one has to look at the whole context of things; that is to say, his data are not anti-vaccine data. His data relate to the possibility that vaccines have effects beyond the specific disease that they're designed for.

Q: So you agree with his findings regarding live vaccines?

A: I agree because, as I've said and as I advised him years ago, that he has to find some immunological correlate to his findings or, otherwise, they're not believable. And what's happened is that scientists not working with Peter have looked at measles vaccination and have shown that the vaccine has effects on what I referred to as natural killer cells before and that they do seem to reduce mortality against other diseases. So, you know, science works that way. One scientist does not gain acceptance for his findings unless they're repeated elsewhere and unless they're consistent with the entire range of facts, not just single ones.

Q: Peter Aaby's a respected researcher, correct? He's a respected researcher, correct?

A: He's a respected researcher. I respect him, just as I respect many other scientists who are attempting to find out things that we don't know yet.

Q: In conducting prelicensure clinical trials for vaccines, what is the difference between solicited and unsolicited reactions?

A: Well, solicited reactions means that you ask the vaccinee whether he's had X, Y or Z. Unsolicited are reactions that the patient reports to the investigator without being specifically questioned about them.

Q: Who decides what gets put on the solicited list and what's -- who decides what symptoms get put on the solicited list of reactions?

A: Well, generally the investigator; however, one has to take into account that the companies meet with FDA during the development of vaccines and that FDA basically has to approve the protocols. And so if FDA thinks that a particular reaction should be measured, they will tell the investigators to include them.

Q: But the list is created by the pharmaceutical company developing the vaccine?

A: In the first instance, yes, and then approved by the FDA.

MR. SIRI: Let's take a two-minute break.

VIDEO OPERATOR: We are going off the record. The time is 11:50.

(Lunch recess.)

Part 3

VIDEO OPERATOR: This is the beginning of Tape No. 3 in the deposition of Stanley Plotkin. We are on the record. The time is 12:37.

BY MR. SIRI:

Q: Dr. Plotkin, earlier you testified that there are two hep B vaccines on the market. One by Glaxo, GSK, that's Endrix-B; and the other one is by Merck, Recombivax HB, right?

A: Yes.

Q: For the Recombivax HB, how long was the safety review period in the prelicensure clinical trial for this vaccine?

A: I don't know.

(Exhibit Plaintiff-10 was marked for identification.)

BY MR. SIRI:

Q: Dr. Plotkin, I'm going to hand you what's been labeled Plaintiff's Exhibit 10. This is the product, the manufacturer insert for Recombivax HB, correct?

A: Yes.

Q: And the clinical trial experience would be found in Section 6.1, correct? Correct? Dr. Plotkin?

A: Yes.

Q: In Section 6.1, when you look at the clinical trials that were done prelicensure for Recombivax HB, how long does it say that safety was monitored after each dose?

A: Five days.

Q: Is five days long enough to detect adverse reactions that occur after five days?

A: No. They would be -.

Q: Is it -.

A: They would be reported separately as observed in the clinic.

Q: In Section 6.1 of the manufacturer insert, which under the Code of Federal Regulations are supposed to describe the clinical trial, does it provide for anything other than five days of monitoring after each dose for adverse events?

A: It does not specifically say that, no.

Q: Okay. Is five days long enough to detect an autoimmune issue that arises after five days?

A: No.

Q: Is five days long enough to detect a seizure that arises after five days?

A: It would be unlikely to have a seizure occur after five days.

Q: Is five days long enough to detect any neurological disorder that arose from the vaccine after five days?

A: No.

Q: Was there any control group in this trial? Let me rephrase that. There's no control group, correct?

A: Not -- let's see. Well, they mention 3,258 doses were administered to 1,252 healthy adults.

Q: That's right. But does it mention any control group, Dr. Plotkin?

A: It does not mention any control group, no.

Q: If you turn to Section 6.2, what is the list of adverse reactions listed in this section?

A: These are reports of adverse reactions that likely were reported to the VAERS system.

Q: Under immune system disorders, does it say that there were reports of hypersensitive reactions, including anaphylactic, anaphylactoid reactions, bronchospasms, and urticaria having been reported within the first few hours after vaccination?

A: Yes.

Q: Have there been reports of hypersensitivity syndrome?

A: Yes. That's what it states.

Q: Does it, reports of arthritis?

A: It is mentioned.

Q: There are also reports of autoimmune diseases, including systemic lupus, erythematosus, lupus-like syndrome, vasculitis, and polyarteritis nodosa as well, correct?

A: Yes. That's what it states.

Q: And also it states that, under the nervous system disorders, it states that after that, there have been reports of Guillain-Barr≈Ω syndrome?

A: Yes.

Q: As well as multiple sclerosis, exacerbation of multiple sclerosis; myelitis, including transverse myelitis; seizure, febrile seizure; peripheral neuropathy, including Bell's palsy;

radiculopathy -.

A: Radiculopathy.

Q: Thank you very much. -- muscle weakness, hypesthesia, and encephalitis, correct?

A: Correct.

Q: Okay. Now, it says at the top -.

A: Before you go on, these reports are required to be included because they have been reported to the authorities as happening after vaccination. That is not proof that the vaccine caused those reactions, because things happen to people all the time, whether or not they've been vaccinated. And as I've said, the company is required to report these. Now, I mention that specifically because multiple sclerosis, for example, is mentioned here. Multiple sclerosis has been studied in relation to hepatitis B vaccine, and there's no relationship, no causal relationship. So the fact that these things are in the package circular does not mean that the vaccine necessarily caused the stated phenomena.

Q: When you say that multiple sclerosis has been studied and is determined to not have been caused, you're talking about the 2011 IOM report, I assume?

A: I'm talking about studies mostly done in France where the situation arose where there was a concern about that.

Q: You're aware of the 2011 IOM report that looked at certain vaccines in relation to whether they can cause certain adverse reactions?

A: Yes.

Q: Are you aware that one of those conditions they looked at was multiple sclerosis?

A: Among others, yes.

Q: Among others. And that they specifically looked at it with regards to hepatitis B?

A: Yes.

Q: And do you know what their finding was?

A: I don't remember the exact wording, no.

Q: Maybe this will remind you: Inadequate to accept or reject a causal relationship. They didn't know, correct?

A: Yes. Yes. But you have to understand, first of all, that science continues and so studies continue. And secondly, that the IOM specifically decided that they would not draw a conclusion if they weren't sure of the conclusion. So what that statement means is that they don't have data that confirm that multiple sclerosis is caused by the hepatitis B vaccine and they, that they don't regard that they have enough data to positively exclude it. So you cannot read that as saying that multiple sclerosis is caused by hepatitis B vaccine.

Q: I never said that. The IOM did for some of the vaccines and adverse reactions, did conclude that it favors rejection of a causal relationship, correct?

A: Yes, that's correct.

Q: But it didn't reach, sorry, it didn't reach that conclusion for hepatitis B and multiple sclerosis, correct?

A: It did not reach that conclusion.

Q: Okay.

A: But other data suggests that that conclusion is warranted, that there is no relationship.

MR. SIRI: Well, I'll make a demand for that. You can produce that after this deposition.

BY MR. SIRI:

Q: What would need to be done to -- in order to know whether or not any of these reported conditions are caused by the vaccine, what you would need is a properly randomized, as you've said earlier, placebo-controlled study, correct?

A: Correct.

Q: Okay.

A: And, also, I would point out that multiple sclerosis is a disorder of adults, and the issue that arose in France was related to vaccination of adults.

Q: Okay.

A: There, that does not mean that it would be an issue, even if it were an issue, for children.

Q: Dr. Plotkin, I was just asking what it says on there. There's lots of conditions listed. I'm not saying that multiple sclerosis is caused by this. I'm just asking if it's listed on Section 6.2. In fact, we can even read the top of Section 6.2 which says: The following additional adverse reactions have been reported with the use of the marketed vaccine. Because these reactions are reported voluntarily from a population of uncertain size, it is not possible to reliably estimate their frequency or establish a causal relationship to a vaccine exposure, right?

A: Correct.

Q: Okay. So that's what it says right at the top of 6.2?

A: Mm-hmm.

Q: But these are events that are reported after vaccination. And as you've just, we just discussed, in order to establish whether it's causal between the vaccine and the condition, you need a randomly, a randomized, placebo-controlled study?

A: Yeah.

Q: But that was not done for this hepatitis B vaccine before licensure, was it?

A: No.

Q: Okay. And given that the vaccine now appears on the CDC's recommended list, isn't it true that it would now be considered unethical to conduct such a study today?

A: It would be, yes, it would be ethically difficult.

Q: So let's take a look at Engerix-B. That's the other the hepatitis B vaccine that you testified that you recommend Faith receive. Do you know how long adverse reactions were reviewed after each dose of that vaccine in the prelicensure clinical trial?

A: Not offhand, no.

(Exhibit Plaintiff-11 was marked for identification.)

BY MR. SIRI:

Q: I'm going to hand you what has been marked Plaintiff's Exhibit 11. This is the manufacturer insert for the Engerix-B, correct?

A: Yes.

Q: Okay. If you turn to Section 6.1, which is clinical trials experience, can you please tell me how long the safety review period was in the prelicensure clinical trials after each dose?

A: All subjects were monitored for four days post administration. That does not necessarily mean that they didn't collect reactions after four days.

Q: Are you claiming they collected reactions after four days but didn't disclose it here in violation of the Code of Federal Regulations?

A: I daresay that they collected putative reactions for a longer period. I feel quite positive about that. When they say they were monitored for four days, that means active monitoring as opposed to collecting reports later on. That is not uncommon in clinical trials.

Q: Is four days long enough to detect an autoimmune issue that arises after four days?

A: No.

Q: Or a neurological disorder that arises after four days?

A: No. That would be reported later.

Q: Uh-huh. And can you provide any proof that there was any reports or follow-up after those four days?

A: Well, it doesn't say that here, but I am willing to bet that they did collect reactions after four days. And I imagine that the FDA would not have allowed them not to do that.

Q: But as you sit here today, that's just speculation, correct?

A: Yes, that's speculation based on experience.

MR. SIRI: I'm going to make a request for you to provide proof of what you're claiming, that there was actually, for both hepatitis B vaccines, any safety review that occurred after four days of administration of any dose of these vaccines.

MS. NIEUSMA: Again, I'm going to continue the objection, I guess, from last time since we took a longer break. There's a proper procedure to request documents in discovery. He doesn't have to come back and produce it.

MR. SIRI: Objection's noted. Thank you .

BY MR. SIRI:

Q: So, and there's no, there was no placebo group, correct? In the 13,000, in the trial at the top where it talks about 13,000 doses being administered.

A: It does not say that there was a control group. I don't know. I'd have to go back and look at the study.

Q: And do you believe, so you think there -.but you're just speculating that there might have been a control group?

A: There well might have been. It's not unusual for controls to be included, especially if you're looking at reactions. But I don't know specifically for this study.

Q: If you're claiming there might have been a control group, then please do provide support for that, because as far as I understand, the manufacturer -- and this was -- who makes Engerix-B? Glaxo? One of your clients. If there was a control group, they needed to have disclosed that. And I assume they're not disclosing it because there was none.

A: Well -.

Q: Go ahead.

A: All right.

MS. RUBY: Go ahead. Ms. Nieusma, are you still there?

MS. NIEUSMA: Yes. My headset died, but I called back in. So I didn't -- I don't think I missed much. Are you still going over the insert?

BY MR. SIRI:

Q: So let's go back to section, now Section 6.2 on this manufacturer insert for Engerix-B. It talks about the post-marketing experience for this vaccine. This one lists for immune disorders, immune system disorders that were reported, a whole number of them, correct?

A: Mm-hmm.

Q: And it also lists a number of nervous system disorders, including encephalitis, encephalopathy, migraine, multiple sclerosis, neuritis -.

A: Mm-hmm.

Q: -- neuropathy, paresthesia -- I'll ask the question all the way at the end. Guillain-Barre syndrome, Bell's palsy, optic neuritis, paralysis, paresis, seizures, syncope, and transverse myelitis, correct? It lists all of those?

A: Yes.

Q: Okay. But to know whether or not these are actually caused by Engerix-B, again, you would need a properly randomized, placebo-controlled study, correct?

A: Correct.

Q: But this study wasn't done prelicensure for this vaccine, right?

A: I'd have to go back and look at the original studies. But these data, undoubtedly, refer not only to the study that was done before licensure, but also to phenomena reported after licensure.

Q: That's 6.2. Okay. And, again, given this vaccine now appears on the CDC's recommended list, it would be unethical to do a randomized, placebo-controlled study of this vaccine, right?

A: In children it would be unethical. It could be done in adults.

Q: Now, if you please go to page 11 of this same manufacturer insert for the hepatitis B, if you take a look over there, I think you'll find that it provides that there was a follow-up with regard to efficacy, not safety, efficacy, that was beyond the four days?

A: Yeah.

Q: Do you see there was a 12-month and an 18-month follow-up?

A: Yes.

Q: So just to be clear, efficacy of the vaccine was followed up for at least 12 months or 18 months, but safety was only done for four or five days?

A: I do not agree with that statement.

Q: Okay.

A: I do believe that GSK, like any other company, would have followed their patients much longer than four days and would have collected reaction data.

Q: And if they didn't do that, you would agree that that is completely inadequate in terms of assessing safety prelicensure?

A: I would say that would be inadequate, yes.

Q: Do you agree with the CDC's recommendation that babies receive a hepatitis B on the first day of life?

A: Yes.

Q: And these are, the Engerix-B and Recombivax HB are the only two hepatitis B vaccines approved for one-day-old babies, correct?

A: Correct. "And why is that?" you may ask. It is because if the baby is not vaccinated -.

Q: I didn't.

A: Well, I'm telling you that if the baby is not vaccinated at one day of age, transmission may occur from an infected mother. And the hepatitis B occurring in babies is likely to become chronic and to cause serious disease later in life. That's why the dose is given at one day of age.

Q: I'm not, I wasn't asking you any questions about efficacy or why it's done.

A: I'm telling you that's why it's given.

Q: Thank you. But, obviously, I'm just trying -- like any product, obviously, you want to have informed consent to understand the risks and benefits. I'm just trying to understand what was done prelicensure for these vaccines. I think you've explained that to me. One of the things you said in the past and I believe is that without clinical trials, without a control group in a clinical trial, you're in la-la land, right? You said that one time? Do you recall?

A: Without a control group, if you're looking for a phenomenon occurring in the vaccine group, you cannot judge that phenomenon without having a control group.

Q: There's only one standalone polio vaccine currently licensed in the United States, correct?

A: Well, as far as licensure, I think both oral and inactivated vaccines are licensed. But the only one that is used in the U.S. currently is the inactivated one.

Q: IPV?

A: Yes.

Q: Right. And there's only one company --Sanofi, there's only one, IPOL by Sanofi?

A: Yes.

Q: A vaccine -- strike that. How long was the safety review for each dose of IPOL in the preclinical trials for that vaccine?

A: I do not know offhand. But, Counselor, IPV has been used throughout the world for years in millions of people, and safety data have been collected on many such studies. And essentially, serious reactions to IPV are extremely rare. So IPV is a very safe vaccine.

Q: I'm asking you in the prelicensure clinical trial for -.

A: That goes back to Jonas Salk where he -.well, he, where millions of children actually were vaccinated with IPV back in the '50s.

Q: And is there clinical trial data on safety?

A: Yes.

Q: Is that the same vaccine that's used today?

A: Yes.

Q: Are you prepared to produce that clinical data?

A: Those data are in this book, and I'll be glad to provide you with the references if you really insist. But IPV, as I've said, has been used in millions and millions of people.

Q: If it's so safe, then how come the safety review period for the prelicensure clinical trial as provided in the manufacturer insert for IPOL only reviewed safety for 48 hours?

A: Once again, I have no doubt that safety observations were made after 48 hours, but they expected that immediate reactions, such as a sore arm or fainting or something like that, would have happened within 48 hours. And, also, I'm sure that they're talking about their own specific production of IPV and not relying on the millions of other people who have been vaccinated with IPV.

Q: I'm going to hand you what's being marked as Exhibit 12. This is the manufacturer insert for the IPOL polio virus vaccine inactivated.

(Exhibit Plaintiff-12 was marked for identification.)

BY MR. SIRI:

Q: If you could please turn -.

A: So let's -.

Q: -- to Section 6.1, Dr. Plotkin. This is an older one. If you could turn to the adverse reactions, which is on page 12, 14.

MS. NIEUSMA: I'll preserve the objection. To my understanding, Dr. Plotkin had no role in study design. You're asking him to speculate as to the reasoning of other people that he had no contact with.

MR. SIRI: Okay. He's testifying that my client should receive this vaccine. I can certainly ask him about the prelicensure clinical trials that were done to assess its safety. And you've put him up as an expert in vaccinology. But your objection is noted and preferred for the record. Thank you, Counselor .

BY MR. SIRI:

Q: Okay. So if you go to page 14, Dr. Plotkin, how long does it say that adverse reactions were observed after vaccination?

A: Forty-eight hours.

Q: Okay. And did the subject group that received IPV only receive IPV or did they receive another vaccine along with it?

A: Concurrently with DTP.

Q: And what did the control group receive?

A: I don't see that stated.

Q: If DTP is given along with IPV, how could you know whether a reaction was caused by DTP or IPV?

A: You could not.

Q: Okay. If you -.

A: However, they do say these systemic reactions were comparable in frequency and severity to that reported for DTP given alone without IPV.

Q: And DTP was the vaccine we talked about earlier that was withdrawn from the market, correct -.

A: Yes.

Q: -- for safety issues? The only MMR vaccines available in the United States are made by Merck, correct?

A: Correct.

Q: How long was the safety review -- do you know how long the safety review period for each dose of MMR in the prelicensure clinical trials for this vaccine? Do you know how long the safety review period for each dose of MMR in the prelicensure clinical trial was for this vaccine?

A: Not offhand. The vaccine has only been used now for about 50 years. Q So it's more recent, right?

A: (No response.)

Q: Dr. Plotkin, I'm going to hand you what's been marked as Plaintiff's Exhibit 13.

(Exhibit Plaintiff-13 was marked for identification.)

BY MR. SIRI:

Q: This is the manufacturer insert for MMR II, correct?

A: Yes.

Q: If you go to the precaution section, I'm sorry, the adverse reaction section, I apologize, on page 6, what you'll find is that there was no clinical trial prior to licensure for MMR, correct?

A: I doubt very much that's the case.

Q: You're not aware that it's -- is it -- are you aware that it is a grandfathered product?

A: I am not aware that it's grandfathered. I was alive and well when the product was first licensed, and it was tested extensively before it was licensed.

Q: So -.

A: So to say that it hasn't been tested is absolute nonsense.

Q: How come there's no clinical trial data in the manufacturer insert?

A: That is something that the FDA would have decided isn't necessary.

Q: Are you willing to -.

A: But we're talking about a vaccine that's been given to millions of children. And just -- I insist on this point, that measles is now a relatively rare disease in the United States because most children receive measles, MMR vaccine. However, in the last, since 2000, because of children who have not been vaccinated, there have been five cases of measles -- I'm sorry, 24 cases of measles encephalitis and three deaths caused by measles itself. So -.

Q: Dr. Plotkin, we'll get to that piece of this, but right now I'm trying to talk to you about the prelicensure clinical safety -.

A: What I'm telling you is millions of doses -.

Q: I understand that.

A: -- have been used of this vaccine -.

Q: I understand you want to -.

A: -- and that there was prelicensure trials -.

Q: Okay.

A: -- which I am absolutely confident about.

Q: Okay.

A: You're talking about stuff that's in a package circular that the FDA has approved and full knowledge that safety and efficacy have been demonstrated.

Q: So you're saying there were clinical trials before the MMR was licensed -.

A: Absolutely.

Q: -- is that correct? And can you provide those?

A: You can find them in this book, if you wish.

Q: So you're saying you won't provide them?

A: Well, yes, I guess I am saying I won't provide them. If you want to take the trouble, read the book.

Q: Sitting here today, when did these, can you tell me what year these clinical trials occurred?

A: Yes. Yes. They were done in the 1960s and the 19 -- yes, mainly in the 1960s.

Q: So you're claiming something happened, but you're not willing to provide any proof that it happened?

A: The proof is in the publications which you can read -.

Q: Can you please turn to the page where it's in there?

MR. SIRI: I'd like to note for the record that Dr. Plotkin has been reading from his notes as well as looking through a book entitled Plotkin Vaccines, Seventh Edition.

THE WITNESS: So on pages -- let's see. Between pages 592 and 600, including tables that show the antibody responses, proportion of children with fever and rash after measles vaccine, et cetera, and the numerous references which go with this chapter.

BY MR. SIRI:

Q: So which, are you saying that that was a prelicensure clinical trial -.

A: Yes.

Q: -- that you just read from?

A: Yes. But, again, I insist the prelicensure or post licensure, the fact remains that the vaccine has been studied extensively over a period of 50 years.

Q: I know -- I understand you want us to just take your word for it, but I prefer to rely on science, peer-reviewed publications and clinical trials.

A: That's what you'll find in there.

Q: So, you know, I understand that you're getting a little upset about me trying to ask for the data, but that's -- I'm just trying to get to the substance. The FDA requires a clinical trial be on the insert. They're not here. Okay? So let's -- you're saying that this table -- and let me take a look at it. This would have been post licensure, not prelicensure. And it doesn't indicate a placebo group, nor that it was -.so I'm not -- this is not a clinical trial, as far as I can tell. Do you have a, can you point me to something that had a placebo group and was prelicensure, please, sir?

A: I'm not sure of the placebo group. I would have to go back and look at the individual studies. But in terms of prelicensure studies, I am absolutely certain that they were done when the measles -- the rubella vaccine I developed was incorporated into MMR. Obviously clinical trials were done before licensure. I'm absolutely certain about that.

Q: Well, maybe they're not included because they didn't include a placebo group.

A: They may not have included placebo group, yes.

Q: So maybe they weren't deemed valid enough to consider a clinical trial?

A: That's absolutely false because you can certainly collect reactions in individuals who receive the vaccine, for example, fever and seizures and that sort of thing that happen immediately and whether there's an effect on blood cells, et cetera. Those things were definitely done. I'm absolutely certain about that because I was there.

Q: But there was no control group?

A: I don't remember there being a control group for the studies that I'm recalling.

Q: So you don't, so you're not aware of any trial that assess safety in MMR with the control group, correct?

A: I cannot cite such a study offhand. I'd have to go back and look to see whether control groups were included.

Q: I'm just, we've, we talked earlier that to assess safety, you need a randomized, placebo-controlled study. And my understanding from looking at this insert is that no such study exists. You told me that it's in this chapter, and you assured me it's in there. But you're not citing to anything in there right now. So I'm happy to get a copy from you if you like to provide it after this deposition. Would you like to do that?

A: I will look.

Q: Going back to page 6, there are, of the manufacturer insert for MMR, there is an extensive list of adverse reactions that have been reported after licensure of this vaccine by individuals receiving the vaccine, correct?

A: Yes.

Q: I'm not going to read through all the ones in the -- because it's a page and a half long, but they're extensive. And, of course, we won't know whether or not MMR actually causes any of these unless we have a randomized, placebo-controlled study, correct?

A: Correct.

Q: When I say "these," I mean all the adverse reactions listed in the manufacturer insert for MMR on pages 6, 7, and 8, right? You understood that's what I meant?

A: Yes.

Q: Okay.

A: Umm -.

Q: Let me ask you this. Listen, let me ask you this. Maybe you can help clarify, okay? You know what? I'll leave that alone. You also testified that Faith should be vaccinated for Hib, correct?

A: Yes.

Q: Okay. Do you know how long the safety review period was for each dose of ActHIB in the prelicensure clinical trials for this vaccine?

A: Not offhand, no.

(Exhibit Plaintiff-14 was marked for identification.)

BY MR. SIRI:

Q: I'm going to hand you what's been marked as Plaintiff's Exhibit 14, Dr. Plotkin. This is the manufacturer insert for ActHIB, correct?

A: Yes.

Q: If we go to Section 6.1 which is the clinical trials experience, I believe you'll see it addresses a number of clinical trials that were performed, correct?

A: Yes.

Q: What were the safety review periods in these trials?

A: Forty-eight hours. Yes.

Q: Actually, you know, if you turn to page 8, Dr. Plotkin, they did one that actually was 30 days long, correct?

A: Say again.

Q: I said if you turn to page 8 of the insert, one of the clinical trials they did actually did look at, did do a 30-day follow-up, correct?

A: Yes.

Q: Now, I'm going to read you a sentence from the paragraph at the bottom of that page. It says: In study P3206, within 30 days following any dose, one through three of DAPTACEL plus IPOL plus ActHIB vaccinees, 50 of 1,455 -- that's 3.4 percent -- participants experienced a serious adverse event, right?

A: Yes.

Q: Now, one way to establish whether or not those adverse events were related to the vaccine was to have a placebo group, a control group receiving an inert substance, correct?

A: That's one way.

Q: That's right. But there wasn't a control group here receiving an inert substance, correct?

A: As far as it says, no.

Q: Right. And the control group here received other vaccines, correct?

A: Yes.

Q: And -.

A: Well, actually, it does appear to be -.well, for dose four, anyway -- oh, no, I'm sorry. Excuse me.

Q: Yeah. It's... It's all right. Anyway, so since there is no placebo group receiving an inert substance, then it's left to the vaccine manufacturer seeking licensure to determine whether or not the 50 -- the adverse events that arose are or are not related to the vaccine, correct?

A: Generally speaking, studies organized by manufacturers or anybody else, for that matter, of vaccines has a safety Board attached to the study. And they evaluate whether they think the reaction was due to the vaccine or not. As it says here, only one of the serious adverse events was attributed to the vaccine, which was a seizure with apnea occurring on the day of vaccination after the first dose, which is, you know, in 7,000 infants and a vaccine that prevents meningitis and other serious diseases is not too bad.

Q: Let's look at that more carefully. This is out of the, out of 1,455, correct?

A: Yes.

Q: And it was 50 children that had a serious adverse event within 30 days, correct? And this -.

A: They had -- let's see. Where is that?

Q: That's the bottom of page 8.

A: Yes. But you have to understand what is meant by "a serious adverse event." They try to accumulate all things that happen to children in a trial. And when they say it's serious, they mean it's not something like pain in the arm or something that's relatively trivial. And then they evaluate whether or not the serious adverse events could be related to the vaccine or not. And what this says is that only one of those events was attributed to the vaccine.

Q: That's right. That's exactly what this says.

A: Yes.

Q: And you told me that the people that evaluate that is a Board set up by the company, the pharmaceutical company seeking approval, correct?

A: Yes. They set up the Board, and they choose individuals who are not employees of the company.

Q: But they choose the individuals, correct?

A: They choose the individuals, yes.

Q: Okay. In your experience, Dr. Plotkin, in any given 30-day period, do 3.4 percent of children in this country experience a serious adverse event?

A: Yes. That's quite possible.

Q: In your experience, would you expect 3.4 percent of children receiving a saline injection to experience a serious adverse event within 30 days of receiving the injection?

A: That's what that means; yes.

Q: Okay. So 3.4 percent every month, that would mean within three years, every child in this country would experience a serious adverse event, correct?

A: Yes. That's correct.

Q: Okay.

A: But you have to understand that "serious adverse events" mean, for example, that a child develops a respiratory infection during the period of the trial. And then the question is, could that respiratory infection be attributed to the vaccine? And the Board decides whether or not it's likely that a vaccine could cause a respiratory infection two or three weeks after the vaccination, for example.

Q: Wasn't there recently a study out of Hong Kong in which it was actually one of the few randomized placebo-controlled studies in which some children were, randomly got flu vaccine and others didn't get the flu shot; and those that got the flu shot and those who didn't had the same rate of flu. But those who got the flu shot were four times more likely to get certain other respiratory infections?

A: I have not read that particular study.

Q: We can get to it later.

A: But influenza vaccine is a whole story in itself.

Q: Okay. That's fine. If you haven't read it, that's, you know, we can get to it. I have it. We'll come back to it. Now, there was, there's another Act, there's another Hib vaccine called Hiberix, right, and then -- which was licensed after ActHIB, correct?

A: Yes.

Q: And in that clinical trial, they used ActHIB as the placebo to assess safety, correct?

A: If you say so.

Q: Okay. The CDC's pediatric schedule, you testified earlier, also includes vaccination for HPV, correct?

A: Yes.

Q: I'm going to hand you what's been marked as Plaintiff's Exhibit 15.

(Exhibit Plaintiff-15 was marked for identification.)

BY MR. SIRI:

Q: Sorry. Handing it to you. This is the manufacturer insert for GARDASIL, correct?

A: Yes.

Q: Which is a vaccine against HPV?

A: Yeah.

Q: GARDASIL is currently the only HPV vaccine used in -- GARDASIL, I'm going to ask you a question unrelated to what I just handed you for a moment while my co-counsel here sends a copy to opposing counsel.

MS. NIEUSMA: You can keep going. I have seen the GARDASIL inserts.

MR. SIRI: Okay. Thank you .

BY MR. SIRI:

Q: So GARDASIL is currently the only HPV used in the United States, correct?

A: I'm not sure whether the GSK vaccine is still being used or not, but GARDASIL is the one that is used mostly in any case.

Q: Can you please turn to page 8, table nine, of this insert.

A: (Witness complies.)

Q: Okay. This table reflects girls and women nine through 29 years of age who reported an incident condition potentially indicative of a systemic autoimmune disorder during the clinical trial, correct?

A: Yes.

Q: The subjects receiving GARDASIL show a rate of 2.3 percent. All right. So that means 2.3 percent of the girls and women in the clinical trial during a six-month period had an incident that indicated a systemic autoimmune disorder, correct?

A: Yes.

Q: Okay. And in the AAHS control or saline placebo group, it shows the same rate, correct?

A: Yes.

Q: Do you know how many individuals were in the saline placebo group versus the AAHS control group?

A: Well, it says 9,412.

Q: That would be the total number for both groups, correct?

A: No. For the placebo group.

Q: For the placebo group, correct. But some of them received AAHS, and some of them received a saline injection, correct?

A: Correct.

Q: Okay. Do you know how many received a saline injection over an AAHS injection?

A: Don't know.

Q: Okay. Let's go to page 4, and table one is for girls and table two is for boys. I'm assuming all participants were either girls or boys. If we add up the saline placebo group for the girls and the saline placebo group for the boys, do we get 594?

A: Well, I have to do the arithmetic. But it appears that there were about 5,000, more than 5,000 in the AAHS control and about 600 in the saline placebo.

Q: Right. It's about 594. It's about 600. That's right, right?

A: Mm-hmm.

Q: Okay. So if we go back to page 8, the saline placebo group had about five in 600, and the rest of them were AAH control, correct?

A: Apparently, yes.

Q: Yeah. What does AAHS stand for?

A: The aluminum adjuvants.

Q: And I see it's defined here as amorphous aluminum hydro -.

A: Hydroxyphosphate sulfate.

Q: Right?

A: Yes.

Q: Thank you. Which we'll refer to as AAHS or the aluminum adjuvant?

A: Yes.

Q: Good? Okay. AAHS is not an inert substance, correct?

A: Well, it's not saline, if that's what you mean. But they use it as a control because they're trying to make, to determine what the reactions are to the HPV vaccine that contains the aluminum and separating the reactions to vaccine from reactions to the aluminum.

Q: Let me try and understand that. Are you saying they're trying to determine what the rate of reactions is between the group that gets GARDASIL -.

A: Yes.

Q: -- with the group that gets the aluminum -.

A: Yes.

Q: -- with the group that gets saline?

A: Yes.

Q: So they want to compare between those three distinct groups, correct?

A: Yes. Mm-hmm.

Q: Okay. And they did do that in table one and two that we just looked at on page 2 -.

A: Yes.

Q: -- page 4, correct?

A: Yes.

Q: Why is aluminum added to the GARDASIL vaccine or any vaccine?

A: To increase the immunogenicity of the active part of the vaccine.

Q: If I may, what you mean is that, if I could use a little more laymen terms, are you saying it's intended to stimulate the immune system to create antibodies?

A: Yes.

Q: Would that be correct?

A: Yes. Not by itself, but by enhancing the response to the vaccine antigens. Q The antigens bind to the aluminum?

A: Yes.

Q: And the aluminum is persistent?

A: Yes.

Q: And it remains in the body such that it continues to present the antigen such that antibodies can be created to it, correct?

A: Well, at least during the immediate period of vaccination, yes.

Q: Okay. There is, in fact, a syndrome called autoimmune/autoinflammatory syndrome induced by adjuvants, correct?

A: That is a debatable point. There's a fellow named Yehuda Shoenfeld, an Israeli, who has pushed this idea for many years, as I think it's fair to say that he has never had acceptance by the larger community of immunologists or rheumatologists.

(Exhibit Plaintiff-16 was marked for identification.)

BY MR. SIRI:

Q: I'm going hand you what is being marked -.I'm going hand you what's being marked as Exhibit 16.

A: Yes.

Q: Are you familiar with this book?

A: Generally speaking, yes. I can't say I've read it all, no.

Q: Okay. And it's entitled Vaccines In Autoimmunity, correct?

A: Yes, correct.

Q: Okay. And it extensively discusses, it's -- it discusses many autoimmune conditions that the authors believe can be caused -.

A: Yeah.

Q: -- by vaccine, and in particular by aluminum adjuvants?

A: I don't know about particularly aluminum adjuvants, but that's one of their arguments.

Q: Can you please turn to the contributors, which starts on Roman, little Roman numeral nine.

A: (Witness complies.)

Q: There are, I think, somewhere around 77 contributors listed here. You said that Yehuda Shoenfeld was kind of alone, I think, or something like that with regard to the claim that autoimmune/autoinflammatory syndrome induced by adjuvants.

A: Yes.

Q: Can you just flip through and look at the universities that are listed here where these over 70 professors hail from. Are these respected institutions of medicine around the world?

A: Well, first of all, Counselor, I have to go over the CVs of each of the people here. You know, I don't know what their role is at the universities. As I said before, Shoenfeld -- first of all, Shoenfeld himself is not anti-vaccination. I know that for a fact. On the other hand, at least one of his co-authors, Tomljenovic, is a well-known anti-vaccination person who has written a lot about how terrible vaccines are. And as far as the articles are concerned, you know, I have to read each one. But, for example, vaccination in patients with autoimmune inflammatory rheumatic diseases, in other words, patients who themselves already have autoimmune diseases, that's a, certainly a legitimate field of study; in other words, how do you vaccinate people who already have autoimmune disease? Could their vaccinations make things worse? But that doesn't necessarily mean that the vaccines themselves cause disease. Now, here we have a chapter called "Measles, Mumps, and Rubella Vaccine: A Triad to Autoimmunity," of which Shoenfeld himself is one of the authors. I am -.what shall I say? I do not believe there is any solid evidence that measles, mumps, and rubella disease cause autoimmune responses. So, you know, lots of books are published, and a lot of them are absolute bull.

Q: Are you saying that this book is bull?

A: I haven't read the whole thing, but I'm almost certain there's a lot of bull in it, judging from the editors.

Q: Without reading it, right?

A: Without reading all of it, yes.

Q: Okay. Are you familiar with the Tel Aviv Sourasky Medical Center?

A: No.

Q: Are you familiar with the University of Paris?

A: University of Paris. Paris has many different universities. They're sort of numbered.

Q: Familiar with University of Pisa?

A: No. I'm sure there is a University of Pisa.

Q: Okay. Are you familiar with the Technion-Israel Institute of Technology?

A: Yes.

Q: The Rappaport School of Medicine?

A: Mm-hmm. I can tell you one thing because I've talked to Israelis about Shoenfeld, and Shoenfeld's opinions are not majority opinions even in Israel.

Q: But for better or worse, there is a syndrome out there that is called autoimmune/autoinflammatory syndrome induced by adjuvants, and there are apparently professors at universities who disagree about the syndrome. But it is out there, right?

A: There is -- Shoenfeld has postulated the syndrome, yes.

Q: And there's at least 70 professors at universities around the world that are in agreement with that syndrome in his book -.

A: No, absolutely not. I'll bet if you go through that book and talk to them, you would find that most of them probably do not agree because all of the articles in this book don't say that vaccines cause autoimmunity. Some of them do.

Q: Okay. There has been concern raised that aluminum adjuvants of vaccines can cause autoimmunity.

A: There has been concerns raised, yes.

Q: Okay. So if there's been concerns raised that aluminum in vaccines can cause autoimmunity and there's this medical text with which I understand your opinion on, why combine the autoimmunity rate in the aluminum adjuvant control with the autoimmunity rate in the saline placebo? Why not break those out to show them separately?

A: Well, they did to some extent. But I think the reasoning was that they wanted to be sure that the reactions that were seen -- and let me parenthetically say that HPV vaccine is painful. And they wanted to be sure that the reactions that they were seeing were not caused by the adjuvant or that they were specific to the HPV antigens themselves and not to the adjuvants. So I can judge that's why they did that.

Q: Well, under that logic, then they certainly should have broken out the aluminum control from the saline placebo control and showed them in two separate columns on page 8, correct?

A: They probably should have, yes.

Q: So that you could see the difference in autoimmune rate between the individuals receiving the aluminum and the saline placebo, correct?

A: Yes.

Q: Okay. In your experience, would you expect 2.3 percent of the girls, of girls and women in this country between the ages of nine and 26 to develop a systemic autoimmune condition in a six-month period?

A: Well, that's a hard question for me to answer. I am not a rheumatologist. But the, when they say "autoimmune conditions," I'd have to read exactly -.

Q: There's a list -.

A: -- what they mean.

Q: If you go to page 8, they've got a long list right there of the conditions. Starts with arthralgia.

A: Right. Yeah. So they have included just about everything that you could consider in autoimmune disorder. And all I can say is that they have, as I -- well, as I've just said, they've attempted to include everything. And those are the data. You know, what can I say? As far as 2.3 percent autoimmune disorders in six months, these are women nine through 26 years of age, so they're not just girls. And I don't think it's impossible that that's the case, especially when you have a list of disorders that is so comprehensive as this.

Q: Okay. So 2.3 percent in six months, 4.6 percent in a year, in ten years half the women in this country would have autoimmunity. In your experience, would that be accurate?

A: Well, again, I am not a rheumatologist, so I cannot answer that question specifically. All that I can say is that they attempted to do a comprehensive study of autoimmune phenomena or putative autoimmune phenomena in this study, and that's what they found.

Q: What, do you know the percentage of girls in the saline placebo group that developed a systemic autoimmune condition during this clinical trial versus the AAH control -.

A: No, I -.

Q: -- AAHS?

A: No, I did not, without going back to the original study.

(Exhibit Plaintiff-17 was marked for identification.)

BY MR. SIRI:

Q: Dr. Plotkin, I'm going to hand you what's been marked as Plaintiff's Exhibit 17. This is the clinical trial data for the saline placebo control group in the GARDASIL trial. You can go to page 2, Dr. Plotkin. You can see that the number of vaccinated in the placebo is 596, right? Or you can see at the top on the first page. I'm sorry. On the first page, Dr. Plotkin, it says: A study of GARDASIL in preadolescents and adolescents, correct?

A: Yeah.

Q: Page 2, you can see this. It has the 596 saline placebo recipients. Can you please turn to the serious adverse event section, which is one, two, three, four, five, six, seven, the seventh page. They don't print with page numbers, unfortunately.

A: Serious adverse events.

Q: Okay. Now, if you go to the next page, one right after that, take a look at that. You can see that the second column is the placebo, the results of the placebo group, correct?

A: Mm-hmm.

Q: Can you please take a minute and go through each page and tell me if there was any value that wasn't zero in terms of finding a serious adverse event?

A: No, I don't see any.

Q: So in the saline placebo group during the trial, there was not a single systemic autoimmune disorder that was reported, but yet there was 218, 2.3 percent, or maybe more actually, in the AAH control when you pull out the saline placebo group. Let me ask -- go ahead, please.

A: Again, you have to do the arithmetic. But if you subtract the 600 or so from the total, you can easily figure out the percentage in the aluminum group.

Q: Right. So let's do that. Let's do that. So there's 900,412 in the aluminum group -- excuse me, in the total, in all of, in both groups combined.

A: Yeah.

Q: If we pull out the saline placebo group of 594 from the 9,412, would that make the 2.3 percent number go up or down?

A: It would go up slightly. That would be -.I'd have to go back and look at the numbers. But that would be reducing the total to about 8800. So I guess that would be in here, right?

Q: Go to page 8.

A: Right.

Q: The point is, is that if they would have broken out -.

A: Two hundred over 8800, and I doubt if that would show a significant difference between the GARDASIL and the AAHS group.

Q: So the GARDASIL group would 2.3, shows 2.3 percent?

A: Yeah.

Q: If we took out the saline placebo group from the second column, it would show 2.3 or above, around 2.3 still, correct?

A: Maybe.

Q: A little higher, 2.4, 2.5?

A: 2.5. Yeah.

Q: 2.5. And then if we had a third column that was just the saline placebo, it would show 0 percent?

A: Yeah.

Q: Wouldn't that have been a significant finding to report?

A: I don't -- you'd have to ask a statistician. But I doubt the statistical difference would be significant.

Q: Doesn't it at least caution having a larger saline placebo group if your concern is statistics in terms of statistical power, which I assume -.

A: Yeah, they might have done that, if they -.

Q: But they didn't do that?

A: Yes. I don't know what that decision was based on. But if you're talking about implication of aluminum, at this point there's really no reason to suspect that aluminum by itself can cause autoimmune disease.

Q: Here's the clinical, prelicensure clinical study in which 2.3 percent of participants in the GARDASIL group and in the control group had a systemic autoimmune disorder, and it was deemed safe because they were around the same rate, right?

A: Yes.

Q: But the saline placebo group that didn't get the aluminum adjuvant had a 0 percent, right?

A: A small group, yes.

Q: Of 594?

A: Yeah.

Q: And so the vaccine apparently -- if you turn back, Dr. Plotkin, to page 4, please of the GARDASIL insert. Are you there?

A: Yeah.

Q: Do you see they break out GARDASIL in one column, those who received AAHS control in another, and those that had saline placebo in a third column?

A: Right.

Q: And that's with only 320 participants in the saline group in table one, correct?

A: Yes.

Q: Okay. And in table two they break it out as well, correct, the saline group from AAHS control group?

A: Yes.

Q: If you turn to page 5, they, again, break out the GARDASIL/AAH control and saline placebo groups in tables three and four, correct?

A: Yes.

Q: But they chose to conveniently combine it when it came to systemic autoimmune disorders, right?

A: Well, in the case of the page 4 and 5, they were looking at local reactions. And, of course, aluminum does give local reactions. On page 8, whether we're looking at systemic autoimmunity, I guess they believed that aluminum in itself is reasonable control and would not cause autoimmunity.

Q: So going into the study, they just assumed aluminum wouldn't cause autoimmunity and so that's how they proceed in designing it. I got it. All right.

(Exhibit Plaintiff-18 was marked for identification.)

BY MR. SIRI:

Q: Dr. Plotkin, I'm going to hand you what's been marked as Plaintiff's Exhibit 18. This is the manufacturer insert for a drug called Enbrel, correct?

A: Mm-hmm.

Q: What is Enbrel a drug for?

A: Well, it's essentially an immunosuppressive, and I think it's used a lot for autoimmune diseases and cancers.

Q: This is a drug given to sick people, not healthy people, correct?

A: Right.

Q: Unlike vaccines which are typically given to healthy children and babies, right?

A: Right.

Q: If you turn to page 10, Dr. Plotkin, all the way to the bottom, the 6.1, Section 6.1, clinical studies experience.

A: Mm-hmm.

Q: The very first line under 6.1 says: The data described below reflects exposure to Enbrel in 2,219 adult patients with RA followed for up to 80 months.

A: Mm-hmm.

Q: So that in studying this drug given to six people, they reviewed safety for up to six and a half years -.

A: Mm-hmm.

Q: -- correct? And they also use -.

(Reporter clarification.)

BY MR. SIRI:

Q: Was that yes?

A: Yes.

Q: And there was, and the placebo group here was, in this study was a saline placebo for all controls, correct?

A: Yes. So what is your point?

Q: I think the point speaks for itself, Dr. Plotkin.

A: It doesn't because Enbrel is given over long periods of time. And one has to, since its immunosuppressive, one has to look for things that may happen because of immunosuppression. Vaccines are given at particular times and are generally not continuously given over long periods of time. But because, aside from that, you're basing this on the package circulars, not on the combined experience with the vaccines that in many cases has taken place over 50 or 60 years.

Q: I'm basing this -- Dr. Plotkin, I'm not basing anything on anything. I'm just asking you questions. And my questions are geared towards being able for my client to be able to pick up what is supposed to be a document that includes the clinical trial experience of the particular biologic or drug and understand what the adverse events rate was for that product. That's all I'm trying to ask you questions about, to understand. That's it. And in terms of your, what you've just said about Enbrel, let's just -- we'll just have one quick vaccine, and then you've really got to move on because I've got a little more material to cover. DTaP vaccine is given at two months of age, correct?

A: Yes.

Q: And at four months of age?

A: Yes.

Q: And at six months of age?

A: Yes.

Q: Eighteen months?

A: Yes.

Q: At three to four years of age?

A: Yes.

Q: And then again at 11 years of age?

A: Yes.

Q: In a slightly DTaP version?

A: Mm-hmm.

Q: So here you have just one vaccine -- put aside the other one -- that is given over an extended period of time. But yet as we saw, as the manufacturer inserts will show, there is no clinical trial that I'm aware of. And I'm happy for you to show me or produce one that actually does what the study in Enbrel does, which is has a saline placebo control group and reviews safety over anything more than, you know, typically a few days or 30-day period.

A: I dispute that. I think it is almost certain, or is certain in my mind, that they observe the patients over a longer period of time, but that they looked specifically for acute reactions during the first few days after immunization. And, also, I add to that, and I insist on repeating that one has to look at the total experience with a drug or a vaccine over a period of time, not simply what is in the FDA package circular.

Q: So are you saying that the, instead of relying on clinical data, saline, inert, placebo-controlled studies, we should just rely on the experience -- well, isn't it true that there's a lot of people out there -- in fact, you've said a lot of, used a lot of adjectives for them today so far -- who are out there and say that their experience is that vaccines have caused all kinds of serious adverse reactions? Isn't that precisely what is on Section 6.2 of each of those inserts? If your approach is used, why are they not given equal weight, I mean, if that's the way we're going to do science? I'm asking for the clinical data.

A: Science depends on a body of work. It does not depend on any single studies. It depends on repetition, on data that confirm other data. And so you cannot take any single study and rely on that and say that is the truth. The truth comes out of repetition and experience.

Q: So is your point just to trust you versus actually have the actual data to support -.

A: No. It's the accumulation of data.

Q: And you can provide data to support everything you're saying here today, correct?

A: Everything that I'm saying is in this book.

Q: You wrote that book?

A: Sorry?

Q: You're the editor of that book, correct?

A: Yes.

Q: It's called Plotkin's Vaccines?

A: Yes.

Q: Dr. Plotkin, what is thrombocytopenia?

A: Decreased platelets.

Q: Can it be caused by an autoimmune reaction? Isn't that what it's known to be caused by, the body attacking its own platelets?

A: That's one of the reasons, yes.

Q: Can the MMR vaccine cause thrombocytopenia?

A: Yes.

Q: What is brachial neuritis?

A: Brachial neuritis is basically a reaction to a local injection where you have pain in the arm.

Q: I'm going to read you a definition of brachial neuritis from Johns Hopkins Medicine, and you can tell me if you agree or disagree with it. Quote: Brachial neuritis is a form of peripheral neuropathy that affects the chest, shoulder, arm, and hand. Peripheral neuropathy is a disease characterized by pain or loss of function in the nerves that carry signals to and from the brain and spinal cord, the central nervous system, to other parts of the body, end quote.

A: Yes.

Q: Can DTaP or Tdap cause brachial neuritis?

A: If it's administered in the incorrect way, yes.

Q: Can the MMR cause febrile seizures?

A: Yes.

Q: Can the flu shot cause Guillain-Barre syndrome?

A: Uncertain, but possible.

Q: Can the DTaP or Tdap cause Guillain-Barre syndrome?

A: Not that I'm aware of.

Q: Hepatitis B cause Guillain-Barre syndrome?

A: Again, I don't think the evidence supports that. Guillain-Barre syndrome is a not-uncommon event, particularly in adults.

Q: After vaccination, is that what you mean?

A: No. I mean in general.

Q: In general. Okay. Can the hepatitis B vaccine cause encephalitis?

A: No, I would say definitely not.

Q: Can the MMR vaccine cause acute or chronic arthritis?
A: It can cause, in adults, it can cause acute arthralgia, I would say, pains in the joints. But that does not seem to be a permanent phenomenon. And it's unusual in children.
Q: So yes for the acute in adults, but otherwise uncertain?
A: In children, it must be quite rare, if it occurs at all. But it does occur in adult women.
Q: Can the flu shot DTaP or hep B cause transverse myelitis?
A: I would say that's unlikely. You said influenza. What did you say, hepatitis B?
Q: Or DTaP.
A: Or DTaP. I think that's the most unlikely.
Q: More likely that it would be the flu shot or hep B?
A: Well, it's difficult with influenza because it is such a widely used vaccine. But I don't see any medical reason why any one of those vaccines should cause transverse myelitis.
Q: But it has been reported?
A: It has been reported. Influenza, I suppose, may be, but I'm not aware of any proof.
Q: Are you aware that -- okay. Can hepatitis B or the flu shot cause fibromyalgia?
A: Fibromyalgia, that's such a vague syndrome. It's, again, difficult to know. But influenza is, there's some differences between influenza vaccine and other vaccines. But with hepatitis B, I don't see any reason why it should cause fibromyalgia.
Q: So no on the hep B and maybe on the flu?
A: Yeah, I guess it boils down to that.
Q: Can DTaP or Tdap cause acute disseminated encephalomyelitis?
A: I would say no.
Q: Can the hepatitis A vaccine cause autoimmune hepatitis?
A: Oh, dear. No.
Q: Can hepatitis B cause lupus?
A: I see no reason why it could.
Q: That's a no?
A: No.
Q: Can influenza cause lupus, influenza vaccine?
A: I can see no mechanistic reason why it would. So I would say no.
Q: Can hepatitis B vaccine cause rheumatoid arthritis?
A: There have been studies along those lines, and I would say that they're unconvincing as far as the vaccine causing rheumatoid arthritis. The difficulty is that rheumatoid arthritis is a common disease. And it, of course, occurs frequently in adults. So it's very difficult to know whether some precipitating event could have caused it. But at this point, I would say no.
Q: Vaccines are also commonly given to most people in the country, correct?
A: They're often given, yes.
Q: So determining causality really requires a double-blind, placebo-controlled study, correct?
A: It does if you want to be certain or at least a statistically strong relationship.
Q: What do you mean by "statistically strong relationship"?
A: I mean a situation where you have a comparative group and you can say that compared to the comparative group, that the association you're looking at is statistically different than the control group.
Q: And from that you believe you can determine causation?
A: Well, you can determine association. Then you have to look and see whether there is

some kind of biological explanation.

Q: Isn't it difficult to determine association -- isn't it difficult to determine an association when it comes to vaccines and an alleged injury because everybody's, for the most part, gets vaccinated?

A: That is true. That is precisely why there are so many false associations between vaccines and disease.

Q: Isn't it also the reason, then, that careful preclinical studies using an inert placebo should be conducted before licensure?

A: It would be ideal to do so. But one would also have to, would have to be very large studies and covering different age groups. And by and large, those data come out much later after experience with the vaccine used in thousands or millions of people.

Q: Well, that, of course, presumes that the, that the adverse events are, long-term adverse events are rare, doesn't it?

A: Yes.

Q: Do you know whether Faith is susceptible to any -- strike that. There's a lot of conditions, so I'm going to try this a little bit of a different way so we can get through this a bit quicker. Is Faith susceptible to suffer any of the conditions we have reviewed thus far?

A: You mean the infectious diseases or the noninfectious diseases?

Q: I'm talking about the adverse event -- I'm talking about the conditions that we just reviewed starting with thrombocytopenia and ending with rheumatoid arthritis.

A: I know nothing about the child and, therefore, am unable to answer.

Q: Do you know whether Faith has a genetic variant that renders her predisposed to suffer any of these conditions from vaccinations?

A: I do not.

Q: Do you know whether Faith has a genetic variance in her microbiome DNA that renders her predisposed to suffer any of the conditions we reviewed?

A: I am not aware of that.

Q: Do you know whether Faith has any environmental exposure that would render her predisposed to suffer any of the conditions that we've just reviewed?

A: No.

Q: In 1991 the IOM issued a report regarding vaccine safety. Are you familiar -- correct?

A: Yes.

Q: Are you familiar with that report?

A: Yes.

Q: That report looked at 22 serious injuries associated with DTaP vaccines and rubella vaccines, correct?

A: Mm-hmm.

Q: Did you provide information to the -- was that a yes?

A: Yes.

Q: Did you provide information to the IOM committee conducting this review?

A: I believe I sent them papers. I was not involved with the committee in any direct way.

Q: Are you aware of whether they thanked you in the introduction -.

A: They may have. I mean, I obviously was a source of information about rubella vaccine, for example.

Q: The IOM searched for evidence regarding whether DPT can cause autism, correct?

A: Yes.

Q: And they could not find any evidence that would help them to make any determination one way or another with regard to whether DPT caused autism, correct?

A: Well, if you mean that they used their statement of not having enough information to make a decision, probably yes.

Q: Do you recall that they had five categories of conclusions, Dr. Plotkin, in that report?

A: Yeah, something like that they had, yeah.

Q: The first category -- strike that. Do you recall that the first category was no evidence bearing on a causal relation?

A: I don't recall specifically, but I believe you're correct.

Q: I'll give you a copy. Let's get you a copy.

(Exhibit Plaintiff-19 was marked for identification.)

BY MR. SIRI:

Q: I'm going to hand you, Dr. Plotkin, what's being marked as Exhibit 19. Dr. Plotkin, the title of this is "The Adverse Effects of Pertussis and Rubella Vaccines," correct?

A: Yes.

Q: By the Institute of Medicine in 1991?

A: Mm-hmm.

Q: Okay. So if we go to, all the way, if we go to the second-to-last page, Dr. Plotkin, I suspect that's what you're looking for. This is a table of the summary of conclusions by adverse event for DPT and MMR, correct?

A: Yes.

Q: So there are five conclusion categories, correct?

A: Mm-hmm.

Q: The first one is no evidence bearing on a causal relation, correct?

A: Mm-hmm.

Q: And what that means, if you see the -- was that a yes?

A: Yes.

Q: Okay. If you go to footnote C, which defines what no evidence bearing on a causal relation means, isn't it true that it says: No category of evidence was found bearing on a judgment about causation. All categories of evidence left blank in table 1-1, correct?

A: Yes.

Q: There's only one condition for which they couldn't find any evidence one way or another on whether it caused, whether the vaccine causes that condition, correct?

A: Right.

Q: And that was -- what was that condition?

A: Autism.

Q: Now, the IOM reviewed whether DPT can cause 17 other serious conditions. And on this chart it found that evidence supported a causation for four of them for DPT; reject a causation for four of them; but that the evidence was insufficient to determine causation for nine of them. Is that correct?

A: Yes.

Q: As for the MMR vaccine, the IOM reviewed four conditions, right?

A: Mm-hmm.

Q: For the first two it -- was that a yes, Dr. Plotkin?

A: Yes.

Q: I hate to trouble you; but if you could say "yes" instead of "mm-hmm," we'd speed things along and I'd appreciate it. For two of them, it found that the evidence was insufficient to make a causation determination, correct?

A: Yes.

Q: But for chronic arthritis, they found that the evidence is consistent with the causal relationship?

A: Yes.

Q: That would be, there's evidence consistent with a causal relationship between the MMR vaccine and chronic arthritis, correct?

A: Yes.

Q: And it also found that the evidence indicates a causal relationship between the MMR vaccine and acute arthritis, correct?

A: Yes.

Q: Do you dispute these findings?

A: Well, first of all, the IOM's later report was not as definitive as far as chronic arthritis is concerned. And the evidence for the consistency, first of all, it must be stressed, we're talking about adults, women, receiving the vaccine, not children. And the other point is that the data really came from one center in British Columbia and was not generally seen. As far as acute arthritis is concerned, it really should be arthralgia, not arthritis, because there's a difference between those two things. But anyway, there's no doubt that the vaccine does cause pains in the joints, but again, particularly in adult women. It is not a big problem in children.

Q: On the next page, Dr. Plotkin, where it says -- of the report, under research needs, does the first sentence say: In the course of its review, the committee encountered many gaps in limitations and knowledge bearing directly and indirectly on the safety of vaccines?

A: Yes.

Q: And then the last says of that paragraph says: Clearly, if research capacity and accomplishment in these areas are not improved, future reviews of vaccine safety will be similarly handicapped, correct?

A: Right. Correct.

Q: Okay.

A: So I think it's worth pointing out that the vaccine community did respond to those conclusions and that, in particular, CDC set up a situation with centers like Kaiser Permanente in California where they do very elaborate safety studies because they have a large, large populations receiving vaccines or not receiving vaccines and they can do comparative studies. And in addition, WHO has set up safety reviews on vaccines. And, of course, CDC has a safety department, and there are funded sort of safety centers throughout the country.

Q: Okay.

A: So it's not as if the vaccine community has ignored the issue of vaccine safety.

Q: Well, wonderful. We'll go through all of that; I can assure you. I've got to take it piece by piece. Okay? So one step at a time. And we will get to Kaiser and the various things that you just talked about. We'll address all of them. I just want to, hopefully we get to everything.

MR. SIRI: You know what? Why don't we take a, just a two-minute, quick break.

VIDEO OPERATOR: I'm going to end the disc.

MR. SIRI: Perfect.

VIDEO OPERATOR: This ends disc No. 3 of the deposition of Stanley Plotkin. We are going off the record. The time is 14:23.

(Brief recess.)

Part 4

VIDEO OPERATOR: This is the beginning of disc No. 4 of the deposition of Dr. Stanley Plotkin. We are on the record. The time is 14:33 .
BY MR. SIRI:
Q: Dr. Plotkin, you earlier said that it would be ethical, you believe, to conduct a randomized, double-blind, placebo-controlled study of the childhood immunization schedule using adults; is that correct?
A: You can't, I suppose you could test childhood schedule in adults; but it wouldn't make a lot of sense, if that's what you mean. You could test individual vaccines, I suppose, although the adults, in all likelihood, will have been either previously vaccinated or previously infected. So it wouldn't be a very easy study to do, but I suppose it's conceivable.
Q: And you think, and it is something that could be done to assess the -- certainly adults are not children. But it would at least give a sense of the safety profile of people who've on the one hand gotten the childhood schedule versus those who haven't. And I would think it's something that you would, you know, any, that you would welcome, given that we should hopefully, I presume, show that both groups will have similar rates of any, of total health outcomes.
A: Well, it's difficult to imagine how one would do it. Now, for example, for hemophilus influenza, disease is rare in adults, of the type B anyway. And so I'm not sure what one would learn by doing such a study. For hepatitis B, of course -.
Q: The adverse events, not the efficacy, Dr. Plotkin.
A: Yeah. Well, I suppose whether it would be translatable from adults to children is uncertain in itself. So I don't think it's a very practical way of studying the safety of vaccines. Fortunately, for hepatitis B, it's indicated for adults as well as children, so that's something that can be done. And papillomavirus vaccine, of course, can be given to adults. So we have data from that type of study. But in terms of systematic studies of childhood vaccines in adults, I don't think that's a very feasible or useful -.
Q: If the group that receives, the adults that receive the full schedule versus those that didn't had significantly higher rates of autoimmune or neurological or other adverse events, you don't think that could provide useful information for potentially making, addressing potential safety concerns and making the schedule safer?
A: So for that you need a group of adults who have never received vaccines.
Q: Why is that?
A: Well, what are you comparing? If you're comparing those who were vaccinated as children with those who weren't, so you need a group that was not vaccinated.
Q: Well, most adults today have not received anywhere near the number of vaccines that children are being exposed to today. So, for example, Dr. Plotkin, you know, when you were a child, as an example, what vaccines did you receive?
A: Diphtheria -- well, in childhood, I think it was probably only diphtheria in those days.
Q: Okay. So if such a study were constructed, would you be willing to participate?
A: You mean as someone who did not receive -.
Q: Yeah. Would you be willing to be part of a study in which you would either, you know,

you would be randomized; you'd either get saline injections or the full childhood vaccine schedule. Would you be willing to do that?

A: Yeah. Well, that -- then you'd have to have -.

Q: I'm sorry. I didn't hear the answer. Would you be willing to do that?

A: Yes. But then you'd have to have a group of 80-year-olds who received all of the childhood vaccines that are now given, which would be pretty difficult to do. So I think this kind of study you're talking about is either difficult or useless because you don't have the right groups to compare. You could do it, perhaps, in 20-year-olds, if you could find 20-year-olds who haven't been vaccinated.

Q: Well, if it was, if they did age controls and so they had a range of ages, including 80- and 20-year-olds, would you be willing to participate?

A: Oh, I'd be willing to participate in any reasonable study.

Q: Okay. Great.

A: But I don't think it would be very useful.

Q: In 1994, the IOM issued another report regarding vaccine safety. Are you familiar with that report?

A: '94?

Q: Yeah.

A: The last one was in the 2000, as I recall.

Q: 2011 was the last one.

A: Okay. Well, there was a large one in about 2000 as well. Anyway, so...

Q: 1994, let me give you...

(Exhibit Plaintiff-20 was marked for identification.)

BY MR. SIRI:

Q: Handing you, Dr. Plotkin, what's been marked as Plaintiff's Exhibit 20. The title of this report is "Adverse Events Associated with Childhood Vaccines," correct?

A: Yes.

Q: This is also by the Institute of Medicine. This is also, in this report the IOM looked at 54 serious injuries associated with a number of different vaccines, correct?

A: Yes.

Q: Okay. Did you provide information to the IOM committee conducting this review?

A: I don't recall doing that.

Q: Do you see on, under the acknowledgments on the second page, your name is in the middle there, Stanley Plotkin, Pasteur, Merieux -- I can't pronounce.

A: Merieux.

Q: Yeah. I don't speak French. I apologize. Can you pronounce that?

A: Merieux.

Q: That's M-E-R-I-E-U-X, C-O-N-N-A-U-G-H-T Company. Now, if you go to, out of these 54 pairs, the IOM found sufficient evidence to support a causal relationship for 14 of them and rejected a causal relationship for four of them. Do you see that?

A: Where are you referring?

Q: So if you go, Dr. Plotkin, to the fourth, fifth-to-last page, it has the causality table.

A: Mm-hmm.

Q: Do you see category three is: The evidence favors rejection of a causal relationship?

A: Yes.

Q: Okay. And you see they rejected it for four of the associated adverse events, correct?
A: Mm-hmm.
Q: Is that a yes?
A: Yes.
Q: You see in category four, it says: The evidence favors acceptance of a causal relation?
A: Yes.
Q: Okay. Do you see that there is, there are five conditions listed there, including Guillain-Barre, brachial neuritis, anaphylaxis. Do you see that?
A: Yes.
Q: And on the next page for category five, which is the evidence establishes a causal relation, do you see that it lists one, two, three, four, five, six, seven conditions, correct?
A: Yes.
Q: Okay. However, for the remaining conditions, so they looked at 54, if we subtract out the three categories we just looked at, 38 of those conditions, the 38 remaining conditions, the IOM couldn't make a causality determination because the science hadn't been conducted yet, right?
A: Yes.
Q: The IOM stated at the end of this report, quote: The lack of adequate data regarding many of the adverse events under study was a major concern to the committee. Presentations of public meetings indicated that many parents and physicians share this concern. Do you see the last page of the report that you're holding of the excerpts? Do you see that it says that on the first two lines under: Need for research and surveillance?
A: Yes.
Q: Dr. Plotkin, in 2011, the IOM then issued its, another report on vaccine safety. And this time it looked at 158 of the most commonly claimed serious injuries after vaccination, right?
A: Yes.
Q: The title of that report is Adverse Effects of Vaccines: Evidence of Causality?
A: Yes.
Q: You're familiar with that report?
A: Yes.
Q: Do you know who commissioned and paid for that report, by the way?
A: Which commission?
Q: I'm sorry. Who commissioned and paid for that report?
A: No.
Q: Would it be surprising to you if I told you that HRSA, the agency within HHS that defends against vaccine injury, claims they commissioned that report?
A: Wouldn't surprise me.
Q: Did you provide information to the IOM committee conducting this review?
A: I don't recall specifically whether I did or not. A lot of people ask for my opinions. When asked, I give my opinions.
Q: Dr. Plotkin, I'm going to hand you what's been marked as Exhibit 21.

(Exhibit Plaintiff-21 was marked for identification.)

BY MR. SIRI:
Q: Is this the 2011 IOM report we were just talking about?

A: Yes.

Q: Do you see there's Roman, little Roman numeral seven, page little Roman numeral seven, see a section entitled Reviewers?

A: Oh, yes. I'm on the list.

Q: Do you see -- I'm going to the first two sentences and can you tell me if that's what this report says. It says: This report has been reviewed in draft form by individuals chosen for their diverse perspective and technical expertise in accordance with procedures approved by the National Research Council's Report Review Committee. The purpose of this independent review is to provide candid and critical comments that will assist the institutions in making its published report as sound as possible and to ensure that the report meets institutional standards for objectivity, evidence, and responsiveness to the study charge. Is that what it says?

A: Yes.

Q: And you're one of the people they gave the report to to review?

A: Yes.

Q: And next to your name, it says: University of Pennsylvania?

A: Yes.

Q: It doesn't disclose that at that time you were working for all four of the major vaccine makers, correct?

A: What do you mean working for them? I mean, at that point I was no longer at Pasteur Merieux Connaught.

Q: In 2011, were you receiving compensation or remuneration from Sanofi?

A: I was, yes, as I've said before. I was consulting for Sanofi as well as others.

Q: Were you consulting for Merck?

A: Yes, probably at that time, yes.

Q: And GSK?

A: Yes.

Q: Okay. And as well as a whole host of other for-profit companies seeking to develop vaccines, correct?

A: Yes.

Q: But I'm just saying, I'm just saying that's not mentioned here, correct?

A: No.

Q: So do you know how many other individuals who were involved in reviewing or compiling this report were receiving money from pharmaceutical companies making vaccines that's not disclosed in this report?

A: I have no knowledge of that.

Q: You provided handwritten comments to the IOM for this report?

A: If I reviewed the report, which apparently I did, I am sure I made comments. I don't know if they were handwritten. Probably not since my hand reading [sic] is illegible.

Q: All right. In this report, the IOM found that 14 of the 158 serious injuries most commonly reported after certain vaccines were, that the evidence supported a causal relationship, correct?

A: Where is that stated?

Q: Well, if you go to page 3 of the report, it's numeral three. Let me ask you the question a different way, Dr. Plotkin. If you look at that chart, you can see that there's little symbols. Do you see those, Dr. Plotkin?

A: Yes.

Q: So an I represents inadequate to accept or reject a causal relationship, correct?

A: Yes.

Q: And an FR means favors rejection of a causal relationship, correct?

A: Yes. Apparently, yes.

Q: If you look through this -.

A: Oh, FA favors acceptance.

Q: I meant -- I said FR. I'm sorry. FR favors rejection.

A: Right.

Q: FA favors acceptance.

A: Mm-hmm.

Q: And CS is convincingly supports a causal relationship, right?

A: Yes.

Q: So I think that, I think what you'll note when you look through this chart is that most of the conditions have an I, correct?

A: Yes.

Q: Any reason -- the report indicates that for 135 out of the 158 reviewed, they found that it could not locate sufficient evidence to make a causality determination, right?

A: Yes.

Q: So the IOM concluded that of the 135 most commonly claimed injuries from vaccination, it didn't know whether or not the vaccines caused that -- let me ask you something. You know, you earlier stated that, you stated that hepatitis B is, doesn't cause encephalitis, right?

A: That's, that's my opinion, yes.

Q: But the IOM, after doing its review, determined it couldn't find science to support a causal determination one way or another, correct?

A: Yes. But that means that they don't have evidence for the supposition.

Q: That it either causes or doesn't cause?

A: Right.

Q: They don't know?

A: They don't know because there aren't enough data.

Q: Okay. But you have -.

A: In the absence of data, my conclusion is that there are no, there's no proof that causation exists.

Q: So if there's no data to show that it causes or doesn't cause -.

A: Yes.

Q: -- your supposition is that -- am I understanding that correctly?

A: Yes.

Q: Is that it doesn't cause it?

A: That there's no proof that it does.

Q: Okay. That's different than saying it doesn't cause it, correct?

A: Correct.

Q: So when you were saying earlier when I asked you at the beginning of this whether certain vaccines caused certain conditions and you said, No, they don't, did you just mean that, no, there's not enough evidence to make a decision one way or another?

A: I mean that there's no knowledge known to me that they do certain things that are, that some may have alleged happen after vaccination.

Q: Like, for example, you know, the IOM reviewed whether hepatitis B can cause lupus because of lots of reports or influenza can cause lupus. They concluded that there's insufficient evidence one way or another to make a determination. You indicated -.

A: Right.

Q: But you indicated earlier that those vaccines don't cause lupus. Your testimony, you're saying that you said no because you weren't aware of a mechanism by which it could cause it; is that right?

A: Yes. That's correct.

Q: Okay. But the science really isn't available to make a determination on causation yet, right?

A: The science doesn't show that there is a relationship. And it is, unfortunately, to prove a negative requires a lot more data than to prove a positive.

Q: If there was a -- I mean, if there was a study that was, had a placebo and a control group, then we could know whether or not these conditions are caused by these vaccines, correct?

A: Yes. It would have to be an enormous study and would have to be randomized ideally, which is unlikely to be the case since -.

Q: It needs to be enormous because you're assuming these conditions are rare, correct?

A: Correct.

Q: Okay. And, and this study that you're saying needs to be done before vaccines are licensed, they do do clinical trials, we've seen, right?

A: Yes.

Q: And they have thousands of people typically in them, correct?

A: Yes.

Q: Okay.

A: And, therefore, they can study common conditions. But uncommon conditions are very difficult to study because they're uncommon; and, therefore, one would need a very, very large study and one would have to have randomization, which is, of course, inherently difficult.

Q: If you actually had a placebo-controlled study, an inert, placebo-controlled study of seven, eight thousand people, you could at least determine that a population of that size, whether or not there's detectable adverse event rate for any of these conditions, correct?

A: For some of those conditions, yes.

Q: All right. I'm going to show you, I'd like to show you an excerpt from that report. Okay? Before I do that, actually, a few quick, little questions. Tdap is one of the vaccines on the childhood schedule, right?

A: Yes.

Q: It's administered to babies during the first year of life?

A: Yes.

Q: We already talked about this at two, four, and six months, right?

A: Yes.

Q: Okay. Did I say Tdap or DTaP?

A: DTaP is the one that's used -.

Q: I meant DTaP. I meant DTaP in that question.

COURT REPORTER: I have Tdap.

MR. SIRI: Okay .

BY MR. SIRI:

Q: Same answer if it was DTaP, correct?

A: Yes.

Q: So let's correct that, please. Now, as for Tdap, T-d-a-p, little d, little a, little p, with a capital T, that's given to pregnant women, correct?

A: Yes.

Q: And DTaP and Tdap refer to vaccines which contain diphtheria toxoid, tetanus toxoid, and acellular pertussis, correct?

A: Yes.

Q: What was the IOM's conclusion in 2011 about whether these vaccines can cause autism?

A: I'd have to look that up, but I feel confident that they do not cause autism.

Q: You feel confident that that's what the IOM concluded?

A: I don't remember what the IOM concluded. But I don't believe there's any evidence that that's the case.

Q: Is there any evidence that that's not the case? Why don't I show you this, Dr. Plotkin.

(Exhibit Plaintiff-22 was marked for identification.)

BY MR. SIRI:

Q: I'm going to hand you what's being marked as Exhibit 22. Oh, Dr. Plotkin, may I actually have that back for a moment. I'm sorry. Nope. I gave you the right one. Here you go. Thank you. This is an excerpt from the IOM's report, right?

A: Yes.

Q: And this is where the IOM discusses the evidence with regard to whether DTaP or Tdap cause autism, correct?

A: Correct.

Q: Okay. If you the turn to the second page, can you read the causality conclusion with regard to whether DTaP and Tdap cause autism?

A: The committee did not identify literature reporting clinical, diagnostic or experimental evidence of autism after the administration of vaccines containing diphtheria toxoid, tetanus toxoid, and acellular pertussis antigens.

Q: Dr. Plotkin, I'm sorry. Can you please read -- Dr. Plotkin, can you please read the causality conclusion with regard to the -- one second, Dr. Plotkin. I'm sorry. The court reporter has to be able to take down the full question or there won't be a clear record. Can you please read the causality conclusion in the IOM report with regard to whether DTaP and Tdap can cause autism.

A: The evidence is inadequate to accept or reject a causal relationship between diphtheria toxoid-, tetanus toxoid-, or the acellular pertussis-containing vaccine in autism.

Q: So the IOM reviewed the available evidence with regard to whether Tdap or DTaP can cause autism, and their conclusion was the evidence doesn't exist to show whether DTaP or Tdap do or do not cause autism, correct?

A: Yes. But the point is that there were no studies showing that it does cause autism except one study by two well-known anti-vaccination figures, Geier and Geier, who have no legitimacy whatsoever. So what they're saying is that there's no evidence. And the important point from my point of view is that there's no positive evidence to do a proper study, as we've been discussing, which would disapprove it, would involve the controlled administration of vaccines and withholding vaccines from children who should have them.

Q: Dr. Plotkin, is there, was the IOM able to identify a single study that supported your claim -.strike that. If you take a look at that section, please, was the IOM able to identify a single study supporting that DTaP or Tdap do not cause autism?

A: No, they did not identify a study.

Q: Okay.

A: But the point is, and I have to repeat myself, that absence of evidence does not allow you to conclude that the two phenomenon are related.

Q: You're making assumptions, Dr. Plotkin, about, I think, what's built -- I understand that. I mean, I only interrupt because, you know, it's 3:00. And I don't mind letting you give a lot of discussion about things that aren't relevant, but to the question -.

A: I think it's relevant in the reports issued by the IOM -.

Q: Yes.

A: -- that their conclusion about evidence not being available -.

Q: Yes.

A: -- does not allow you to conclude that the phenomena, that there is a causal relationship.

Q: I'm not sure -- I never said that. I'm not sure anybody in this room said that, Dr. Plotkin.

A: Good. I like to hear that.

Q: But it does allow you to conclude that the evidence doesn't exist to say that DTaP and Tdap do not cause autism, correct?

A: There is not evidence to say a million different things -.

Q: Okay.

A: -- but you have to prove -.

Q: Did the IOM report look at whether the MMR vaccine can cause autism?

A: I'd have to look and see.

(Overtalking.)

BY MR. SIRI:

Q: Yes -.

A: I believe it did.

Q: -- it did.

MR. SIRI: I'm sorry. He said it did.THE WITNESS: I'm looking to see .

BY MR. SIRI:

Q: It said it favors rejection because it did find studies -.

A: Yes.

Q: -- correct?

A: Yes.

Q: That's right. So studies are possible to determine whether or not a vaccine does or does not cause, does not cause autism, correct?

A: They are possible, yes.

Q: Okay. But the study to determine whether DTaP or Tdap does not cause autism has not been done, right?

A: A study that would definitively show that it doesn't has not been done, but there's no evidence that it does.

Q: But since, Dr. Plotkin, we don't know whether DTaP or Tdap cause autism, right, it would be a bit premature to make the unequivocal, sweeping statement that vaccines do not cause autism, correct?

A: In the absence of evidence, one should not draw any conclusions except that there's no evidence. And so I don't infer from the absence of evidence about a million different things that they're necessarily true. One has to do studies to determine whether or not a phenomenon exists, and usually those studies are done because there's some suspicion that, of a relationship. But in, we have no suspicions, at least I don't, that autism is caused by DTaP.

Q: Well, you may not have that suspicion, but it is one of the most commonly reported conditions, adverse events, which is why it was reviewed in this IOM report from DTaP/Tdap, which we discussed earlier. So I just, I'm not saying, I'm not asking you to say that vaccines do cause autism. I'm not asking that at all. I'm asking you, as a scientist, can you make the statement that vaccines do not cause autism if you don't know whether DTaP or Tdap cause autism?

A: As a scientist, I would say that I do not have evidence one way or the other.

Q: Right.

A: As a practicing physician, I have to weigh all kinds of things in making a decision about a patient, whether to do something or not to do something. And I make that, those decisions based on the body of knowledge, even in the absence of definitive information for every case. This has been true for medicine ever since its inception.

Q: I'm asking you a simple question. I'm asking you, since the science has not yet been done regarding whether DTaP or Tdap cause autism, isn't it true that you cannot make the sweeping statement that vaccines do not cause autism?

A: I can make the statement that there is no evidence that vaccines cause autism, and, therefore -.

Q: I'm not asking you that question -.

A: -- and, therefore, and, therefore -.

Q: -- Dr. Plotkin.

MS. NIEUSMA: (Inaudible.)   It's time to move on.

MR. SIRI: He's not answering the question.

THE WITNESS: -- and, therefore, vaccines should be given to protect against serious diseases.

BY MR. SIRI:

Q: Dr. Plotkin, we've already reviewed the IOM report. The IOM could not find evidence that DTaP or Tdap cause autism. I'm asking you, knowing that, isn't it just a bit premature to make the unequivocal, sweeping statement that vaccines do not cause autism?

A: I would say it is logically true that you cannot say, you cannot point to proof that it doesn't cause autism. But as physicians and public health specialists, one has to make decisions in the absence of thousands of pieces of information that one would like to have. And one of them is that vaccines protect against serious infectious diseases, and there's no evidence that they cause autism. So, therefore, I recommend vaccinations to this child and every other child who does not have a contraindication.

Q: But since there's no evidence that DTaP or Tdap don't cause autism, you can't yet say that vaccines do not cause autism, correct?

MS. NIEUSMA: (Inaudible.)

THE WITNESS: I could not say that as a, as a scientist or a logician. But I can say as a physician that, no, they do not cause autism, because as a physician, I have to take the whole body of scientific information into consideration when I make a recommendation for a child .

BY MR. SIRI:

Q: The IOM reviewed the science. They didn't find a single study that supported whether or not vaccines -. (Discussion off the stenographic record.)

MS. NIEUSMA: At this point, Dr. Plotkin, just wait for him to move on to the next question.

MR. SIRI: I'm not asking the same question, Counsel. Your objection is noted. I'm responding to his comments, which are different every time.

BY MR. SIRI:

Q: So what you're saying is a physician or logician, then, you couldn't say vaccines do not -.you could not say vaccines do not cause autism. But as a pediatrician, you're saying that you would say that to a parent because you want to make sure they get the vaccine; is that right?

A: You know, I can't be sure that DTaP doesn't cause leprosy. That doesn't mean that stops me from using DTaP vaccine.

Q: Are people claiming that DTaP has caused leprosy? Are you aware of any such complaints?

A: I'm not aware of any such complaints, but I wouldn't be surprised to see it on the web one of these days.

Q: Okay. But people have made enough complaints about DTaP, Tdap causing autism that the Institute of Medicine at the commission of HHS thought it was serious enough to do a scientific review, correct?

A: Yes.

Q: Okay. They didn't review whether DTaP causes leprosy, did they?

A: No.

Q: Okay. So, and after conducting that review, they found that there was no evidence at all that they could find whether DTaP or Tdap caused autism. I'm just asking you a simple question, which is since there's no evidence whether DTaP or Tdap cause autism, isn't it a little premature to say, to make the sweeping statement that vaccines do not cause autism?

A: No, I do not agree with that. Because absence of evidence works both ways. There's no evidence that they do, and the ideal study has not been done. I agree with that. But in the absence of any reasonable evidence that they do, I continue to recommend their use.

Q: So you're willing to make a statement that a vaccine does not cause a condition even in the absence of any evidence?

A: I'm willing to state that there is no evidence that the vaccine causes the condition and, therefore -- and there is a lot of evidence that they do protect against disease. And, therefore, the child should receive the vaccines. I mean, there are a million things on the web, including all kinds of diet advice based on ridiculous information. So why should I adopt that?

Q: Are you saying that the IOM was engaging in a ridiculous review here?

A: They were doing a scientific review, which is certainly legitimate. And their conclusion that there are insufficient data to draw a formal conclusion, I can understand that and appreciate that. But that does not mean that the vaccines cause autism.

Q: You've never been asked that. The only thing I've asked you is whether or not one can assert that vaccines do not cause autism, that they do -.

A: Counselor, let's be, let's be real. You're asking me these questions because you want me to legitimize the view that vaccines cause autism, and I will not do that because absence of evidence is no proof whatsoever.

Q: I think that record is very clear, Dr. Plotkin. I'm not trying to legitimize anything. I'm just asking you to, I'm not trying to legitimize that vaccines cause autism. I think I'm very clear

A: I'm glad to hear that.

Q: -- we have very clearly established what the IOM found. The IOM found in their estimation no evidence, right?

A: Right.

Q: They found no evidence that vaccines do cause -- excuse me -- that DTaP or Tdap cause autism. Let's make that very clear, right?

A: Right.

Q: They found no evidence that DTaP or Tdap cause autism -.

A: Yes.

Q: -- period. They found one study which they said was unreliable because it relied on VAERS data and it had no control, right?

A: Right.

Q: Okay. But similarly, in the same vein, they also didn't find any evidence that DTaP/Tdap do not cause autism. Now, that doesn't mean that DTaP/Tdap do cause autism, correct?

A: Correct.

Q: It doesn't mean that, right?

A: Yes.

Q: That's right. All it means is that they couldn't find a study that showed, that supported that it does not cause autism, right?

A: Yes.

Q: Until -- and that's why they reached the conclusion that they did, which is they said the data is insufficient, right?

A: Mm-hmm.

Q: I assume you -- was that a yes?

A: Yes.

Q: Do you agree with the IOM's conclusion that the data, the evidence is insufficient to determine whether or not DTaP/Tdap cause autism?

A: I agree with their conclusion, but that doesn't mean that I don't act on other information.

Q: Okay. Okay. I can understand that. I can understand that. But you make -- I'm not, I'm not saying that -- I'm not asking you to ignore any benefits you believe accrued from vaccines. Okay? I'm not asking you to do that at all, Dr. Plotkin. I'm simply asking you as a pure matter of logic. As a pure matter of logic and common sense, if you don't know whether A causes something, can you say A, B -- let me not use that hypothetical. If you don't know whether DTaP or Tdap cause autism, shouldn't you wait until you do know, until you have the science to support it to then say that vaccines do not cause autism?

A: Do I wait? No, I do not wait because I have to take into account the health of the child.

Q: And so for that reason, you're okay with telling the parent that DTaP/Tdap does not cause autism even though the science isn't there yet to support that claim?

A: Absolutely.

Q: Okay.

A: I'm also willing to tell them it doesn't cause leprosy.

Q: Again, did the IOM review whether DTaP caused leprosy?

A: No.

Q: Okay. All right. Dr. Plotkin, has there ever been a study which looked at the total health outcomes of children following the CDC's vaccination schedule and those who are completely unvaccinated, such as Faith?

A: Not that I'm aware of. No, I don't think so. But, you know, there are all kinds of studies. There's a study that suggests that children who are vaccinated compared to unvaccinated children have lower rates of leukemia. Now, do I believe that study? I find it interesting, but I would want confirmation of that study before I believed it. But just to point out that Peter Aaby, for example, as I mentioned before, found measles vaccination had a positive effect on health and reduced mortality. So I think there is abundant evidence that vaccines do contribute to the health of children. But in answer to your question, there is no study that I know of that compared the health of vaccinated children with unvaccinated children.

Q: Why has that study not been done?

A: Probably because it is considered bad, malpractice not to vaccinate a child.

Q: So you are saying a prospective study might be improper because it would leave a child unvaccinated?

A: Correct.

Q: Okay. What about a retrospective study?

A: That, I suppose, could be done, but it wouldn't be randomized.

Q: When I say "retrospective," that means using existing data, correct?

A: Using -.

Q: Why don't I ask you -- strike that. Can you define "retrospective," please.

A: I mean, looking at children who had been vaccinated and comparing them to children who had not been vaccinated.

Q: Okay. Presumably, HMOs, insurance companies would have health data on enough vaccinated and unvaccinated children to conduct such a comparison, correct?

A: Well, I don't know, because the percentage of unvaccinated children fortunately is quite low. So I'm not sure how easy it would be to do that study. And I would suspect that many of those unvaccinated children are not in registers that could be used.

Q: You're familiar with the Vaccine Safety Datalink?

A: Yes.

Q: Are you aware that there are a few thousand children that are, my -- are you aware that there are reports from the government, government reports that show that there are a few thousand children that are, my understanding, completely unvaccinated in the VSD?

A: Oh, I don't doubt it.

Q: Okay. Couldn't the Vaccine Safety Datalink be used to conduct a retrospective "vaccinated versus unvaccinated" study to look for health outcomes?

A: Well, I don't know. Theoretically, perhaps, but one would have to be convinced that the children were comparable in other ways besides being vaccinated or unvaccinated.

Q: Every time you do a retrospective study, you always need to control for potential cofounders [sic], correct?

A: Yes.

Q: That's what you're talking about, controlling for cofounders, right?

A: Yes.

Q: And, you know, if you're doing a case control, properly matching cases, or if you're -.right? Are you saying that -- so CDC, pharma, they conduct studies all the time, right?

A: Mm-hmm.

Q: Including studies -.

A: Yes.

Q: Yes. Including studies that have cofounders that need to be controlled for, right?

A: Yes, they try, yes.

Q: Vaccine studies, especially for efficacy, happen all the time, correct?

A: Yes.

Q: So, again, if the data is there, why not do a study comparing vaccinated to completely unvaccinated children to look for the total health outcome so you know what the real risks are or get at least a sense of what the real risks are from vaccinations?

A: Well, I can't completely answer that question. I'm sure it would be a difficult study to do. But I will repeat what I said earlier about measles vaccination. I would just remind you again that among those children who were not -.

Q: You've already said all this, Dr. Plotkin. It's fine. I got it.

A: I'll repeat it. There were three deaths and 24 cases of encephalitis. And that's unbearable.

Q: I'm sorry.

MR. SIRI: Can you read back what Dr. Plotkin just said. - - . (Whereupon, the Reporter read back a preceding portion of the testimony as directed: "A. Well, I can't completely answer that question. I'm sure it would be a difficult study to do. But I will repeat what I said earlier about measles vaccination. I would just remind you again that among those children who were not -. "Q. You've already said all this, Dr. Plotkin. I got it. "A. Well, I'll repeat it. Three deaths and 24 cases of encephalitis. That's unbearable.")

BY MR. SIRI:

Q: Dr. Plotkin, who prepared the notes that are in front of you?

A: Me.

Q: Okay. When did you prepare those?

A: Oh, about a week ago, I guess.

Q: During the break, our lunch break, did you talk with anybody?

A: No -- well, yes. I talked with my wife.

Q: Anybody else?

A: No.

Q: Okay. So I understand that you find injuries that can result from what you've called, I believe, vaccine-preventable diseases. What I'm trying to do is understand the risks of vaccinating and, in particular, for Faith. And can you appreciate that, understand -- strike that. So you just think it's too difficult to look at, to do a study comparing vaccinated and unvaccinated children, even though the data exists to do that; is that right?

A: Well, I simply am saying that I don't know how feasible it is. I've never been asked to look at it before, but I do think a priori that it would be difficult because those children are very likely from different socioeconomic groups and different racial groups. And so it would be a different study to do. I don't know if it's feasible or not.

Q: So with all of the government -- so the pharmaceutical industry, you said, made approximately $20 billion last year in revenue from vaccine sales?

A: I think so. I don't have -.

Q: I have the financial statements. Should we review them, or do you think 20 billion is about right?

A: I think it's about right. I'm not an accountant -- I don't make -.

Q: Give or take a few, give or take a billion or two, would you say?

A: I think so, yes.

Q: Okay. So the pharmaceutical industry has $20 billion in revenue, and the CDC spends hundreds of millions of dollars buying vaccines every year; is that right?

A: I think so.

Q: But yet you don't think that the resources can be done to do a single solitary study comparing the health outcomes of a for-profit product given to almost every child in this country to assess what the rate of adverse reactions are between those who get all those products and those who don't?

A: What I said is I simply don't know whether such a study is feasible or not, but I think it would be difficult to do because it would not be a randomized study; and, therefore, the conclusions might be, might be questionable. But I don't know whether such a study is feasible or not.

Q: Aren't most studies that are done that you rely upon in that book that you have in front of you not randomized?

A: Many of them are not. Many of them are.

Q: Do you throw out the ones that are not randomized?

A: It depends on what the purpose of the study is. If it's studying immune responses, it doesn't necessarily have to have a control group.

(Exhibit Plaintiff-23 was marked for identification.)

BY MR. SIRI:

Q: Dr. Plotkin, I'm going to hand you what's being marked as Exhibit, Plaintiff's Exhibit 23. Dr. Plotkin, what is an ICD-9 code?

A: Well, it's essentially a way of coding diseases for, usually for remuneration purposes.

Q: Okay. So when a doctor administers a drug or a diagnosis as a patient or something similar, there's a code that they would enter into the system, right?

A: Yes.

Q: And the ICD-9 codes are published by the American Medical Association, correct?

A: Yes.

Q: Okay. Please take a look at the exhibit I just -- the exhibit I just handed you is the 2015 ICD-9-CM Professional Edition for Physicians codebook, correct?

A: Yes.

Q: Or at least the front page and one excerpt, correct?

A: Mm-hmm. Yes.

Q: So if you go to the second page, do you see there's a code, V6.407?

A: Yes.

Q: What is that code for?

A: Vaccination not carried out for religious reasons.

Q: Okay. So wouldn't it be feasible, for example, to compare children who have this coding who are not being vaccinated with those who are being vaccinated who are in similar communities, have similar demographics, and otherwise avoid as much as possible other potential cofounders.

A: Well, if you could eliminate the cofounders it would be feasible.

Q: What are the cofounders, Dr. Plotkin?

A: Well, as I said before, the cofounders include socioeconomic level, racial grouping, exposure to agents. In other words, are they living in a community where it's unlikely that someone unvaccinated from Ethiopia is going come into the community and be able to transmit diseases? I mean, I'd have to sit down and write up a list of possible cofounders. But there would be many of them.

Q: So when you do studies for efficacy, are you able to control for all of these cofounders?

A: Well, usually the effort is to include as many different types of individuals as possible so that if there is a problem with a particular group, you can identify it. But doing clinical studies is not always easy, and that's why the conclusions from clinical studies have to be seen in relation to other clinical studies.

Q: Why is it you can control for cofounders in various other vaccine studies, including in vaccine safety studies that are cited in your book, but you believe -- are you saying you couldn't control for these same cofounders in the study of vaccinated versus unvaccinated population?

A: I am unable to draw a conclusion about whether such a study is feasible. What I'm pointing out is that the likelihood of there being multiple cofounders is -- confounders, sorry, is very high; and, therefore, it wouldn't be an easy study to do. That's all I can say. I've never sat down to try to figure out how to do such a study.

Q: Well, we've got socioeconomic, which probably pretty easy to control for; racial grouping, pretty easy to control for; exposure to agents, since it's retrospective, you'll know if there's been an outbreak in the community. What other cofounders do you think might exist? I mean, I'd like to hear one that -.can you tell me a cofounder that's not easy to control for?

A: In principle, one can control for any confounding problem. The issue would be just how many there are and just how large a group you would need for a statistical significance. See, that's another issue. I mean, we accept as a valid conclusion something that is false five times out of a hundred. And so not only do we have to try to eliminate confounders, but we also need repetition of studies to be sure that the results we got in the first study were not in the five studies that were false -.

Q: Great.

A: -- in their conclusion. So you would need multiple studies.

Q: Okay. And since these are retrospective, they're really just running data, right?

A: If the data are encoded, yes.

Q: So I asked earlier, what cofounder can you list that's not easy to control for? And I did not hear another cofounder. Can you tell me a cofounder in this proposed study that would not be easy to control for?

A: Exposure would be probably the most difficult; in other words, whether a child is living in a community where exposure to disease is rare or absent or whether the child is living in the community where there are significant possibilities of exposure. I think that would probably be the most difficult to account for.

Q: When's the last case of polio in the United States, wild polio?

A: Oh, I forget the exact year, but it's been probably 20, 25 years.

Q: 1979 sound correct to you?

A: Yeah, could be.

Q: So that wouldn't be an issue, correct?

A: No. Polio would not be an issue.

Q: Okay. How many cases of diphtheria have there been in the last ten years in the United States?

A: It's very rare or absent.

Q: Less than five, right?

A: Yeah.

Q: Isn't that true for most of the diseases except for maybe pertussis, right?

A: Well, pertussis, HIV, hepatitis, those are diseases that are still common.

Q: So if we excluded -.

A: The mumps. Yeah.

Q: Go ahead. Mumps, pertussis. Okay. So since this is retrospective, we would know where those outbreaks are, right?

A: Yes.

Q: Because they're very carefully tracked by the CDC, correct?

A: Mm-hmm.

Q: Since we know where the outbreaks are for those diseases, that could be -- was that a yes?

A: Yes.

Q: Since we know where those outbreaks are, that could be actually probably pretty easily controlled for as well, correct?

A: In principle, yes.

Q: Okay. So can you name me a cofounder that would be difficult to control for in the study?

A: Well, at the moment I can't think of any other that would be material, although I think one would have to look at genetic issues and the health of other members in the family and so forth. But, again -.

Q: Okay.

A: -- I am not saying that such a study is impossible. I'm just pointing out that it would be a very difficult study to do, and the conclusions that you could draw from the study might be very limited.

Q: Well, you keep saying it's difficult. But I, and your reason for that, I understand, is potential cofounders. And I'm just trying to understand what those are. So you've said familial history. Presumably the parents would be in the same health plan as the children. So you have the parents' medical history, too, correct?

A: Mm-hmm.

Q: So that could be controlled for as well, right?

A: Yes.

Q: You said "mm-hmm" two questions ago -.

A: Yes.

Q: -- that was a yes? Okay. So that could be easily controlled for, correct?

A: Yes.

Q: Okay. And so can you tell me again, can you tell me a cofounder that would actually be difficult to control for in this study?

A: Well, other than the ones that I've mentioned and not having thought about doing such a study, that's all I can say.

Q: If you did such a study, isn't it -- are you aware that advocacy groups and other people interested in this issue have been calling for this exact study of comparing vaccinated and unvaccinated for 30 years already?

A: I don't spend a lot of time on the web, so I can't say that I know that such a study is being requested.

Q: Okay. Well, but you do read IOM reports and CDC reports?

A: Yes.

Q: Okay. And you never come across any IOM or CDC reports in which they specifically address the repeated calls for such a study?

A: No.

Q: Okay. Would it be surprising to you if I told you those existed?

A: That what existed?

Q: That CDC and IOM reports in which they document the calls for such a study.

A: Well, I wouldn't be surprised, no.

Q: Would you be surprised to know that the CDC, in fact, issued an entire report regarding conducting such a study and the calls for conducting such a study?

A: And they issue the -- what did you say?

Q: Would you be surprised to know that the CDC, in fact, issued a report in response to the request for the calls for such a study?

A: I wouldn't be surprised that there's a response, no.

Q: Okay. So in looking for such a study, isn't it true that there actually has been one such study conducted in the past, for the first time ever in the last year, correct?

A: I am not aware of that study.

(Exhibit Plaintiff-24 was marked for identification.)

BY MR. SIRI:

Q: Okay. I'm going hand you what's been marked as Plaintiff's Exhibit 24. The title of the study is a "Pilot Comparative Study of the Health of Vaccinated and Unvaccinated 6- to 12-Year-Old United States Children," correct?

A: Yes.

Q: And the authors of this study are Professors at the Department of Epidemiology and Biostatistics, School of Public Health, Jackson State University, correct?

MS. NIEUSMA: Just a minute.

THE WITNESS: That's what it says.

MS. NIEUSMA: Just a minute. (Inaudible.)

MR. SIRI: Absolutely. I'm sorry. Let's just wait for counsel to get a copy.

MS. RUBY: Sorry about that.

MR. SIRI: I thought it had gone. Okay. So -.

MS. RUBY: Ms. Nieusma, do you have it?

MS. NIEUSMA: I should in just a -- yep.

MS. RUBY: Thank you. Sorry about that .

BY MR. SIRI:

Q: Are you familiar with this pilot study, Dr. Plotkin?

A: No. I see it's been published in the Journal of Translational Science, which is not one of the journals I read and is probably one of those multiple so-called predatory journals that we are trying to deal with currently.

Q: So is anybody in any university that publishes anything that's negative about vaccines predatory or -- I forgot the other adjectives you used earlier today.

A: No, it's not, it's not that. It's that there are journals now that will publish anything for money.

Q: Oh.

A: And I get about ten of those invitations a day.

Q: So does money influence judgment?

A: It may.

Q: Conduct?

A: It may.

Q: Okay.

A: I cannot tell until I read this study.

Q: I understand. So, well, in this study, if you look, if you take a quick look at it, you'll see that it involves looking at total health outcomes between vaccinated and unvaccinated homeschooled children?

A: Yes.

Q: When you're ready, please turn to page 5. Do you see the row that says: Chicken pox?

A: Yes.

Q: Okay. So the odds ratio for the unvaccinated were twice as likely -- no. I'm sorry -- four times as likely to get chicken pox, right?

A: Yes.

Q: .26, so odds ratio of about four. The kids who were unvaccinated were about four times more likely to get chicken pox?

A: Mm-hmm.

Q: Okay. Is that a yes?

A: Yes.

Q: And do you see for whooping cough, the unvaccinated children were three times as likely to get whooping cough?

A: Yes.

Q: Go down to where it says: Allergic rhinitis.

A: Yes.

Q: What is that?

A: Well, it's essentially runny nose because of allergy.

Q: Okay. Do you see that it says that the vaccinated children were 30 times as likely to have allergic rhinitis?

A: Yes, I see that number.

Q: Do you see that it says that vaccinated children were 3.9 times likely to have allergies?

A: Yes.

Q: 4.2 times as likely to have ADHD?

A: Yes.

Q: 4.2 times likely to have autism spectrum disorder?

A: Yes.

Q: 2.9 times as likely to have eczema?

A: Yes.

Q: 5.2 times as likely to have learning disability?

A: Yes.

Q: 3.7 times as likely to have neurodevelopment disorder?

A: Yes.

Q: And 2.4 times as likely to have any chronic condition?

A: Yes.

Q: Wouldn't you like to see a larger-scale study that refuted these claims?

A: It would be ideal, yes. It would certainly be important to repeat the study and to enroll patients in a blinded fashion. I really would have to read this to see exactly how they enrolled the children or the parents in this study.

Q: Doesn't the existence of this study, though, I mean -- strike that. So it at least calls for further similar studies, hopefully, to either confirm or disapprove the findings in the study, correct?

A: Yes. Mm-hmm. Yes, I would agree.

Q: I'm going to show you one more study that was done with the same data from this author.

(Exhibit Plaintiff-25 was marked for identification.)

BY MR. SIRI:

Q: Dr. Plotkin, I'm going to hand you what's been marked as Plaintiff's Exhibit 25. This is another study by the, this is another publication using the same data, I believe, from the same group of professors at the Department of Epidemiology and Biostatistics School of Public Health, Jackson State University, correct?

A: Appears that way, yes.

Q: And the title of this one is "Preterm Birth Vaccination and Neurodevelopmental Disorders: A Cross-Sectional Study of 6- to 12-Year-Old Vaccinated and Unvaccinated Children," correct?

A: Yes.

Q: I'll give you a moment to read the abstract. Have you ever seen this study before?

A: No.

Q: Okay. So just take a moment, please, and read the abstract.

A: Mm-hmm. Yes.

Q: So in the middle of the abstract, I'm going to read two sentences. And you can tell me if I've read them correctly. No association was found between preterm birth and NDD in the absence of vaccination -- strike that. Actually, Dr. Plotkin, one, two, three, four, five, six, seven lines down in the abstract, do you see where it starts: No association?

A: Yes.

Q: Can you start, can you read that sentence and the next one?

A: No association was found between preterm birth and NDD in the absence of vaccination, but vaccination was significantly associated with NDD in children born at term. Odds ratio, 2.7. Is that sufficient?

Q: you.

A: And the next sentence, please, sir. Thank However, vaccination coupled with preterm birth was associated with increasing odds of NDD, ranging from 5.4 compared to vaccinated, but non-preterm children to 14.5 compared to children who were neither preterm nor vaccinated.

Q: What does NDD stand for?

A: Neurodevelopmental disorders.

Q: And in this study it was defined as learning disability, attention deficit hyperactivity disorder, and autism spectrum disorder, correct?

A: Yes. But I will also point out the abstract says that it was a convenient sample of 666 children. So clearly it was in no way a randomized study.

Q: Shouldn't we do better studies?

A: One would have to do a better study if -.

Q: Larger samples?

A: Larger samples and enrolling not by convenience.

Q: Right. I believe Dr. Mawson calls these pilot studies, correct? Because nobody else is doing them, so he tried with limited resources, not the resources of pharmaceutical companies and the CDC, to conduct such a study, right?

A: Well, that's your interpretation. I would have to read the study.

Q: Fair enough. More than fair. Is it possible that his findings in both of these studies could be correct?

A: Is it possible? Yes, of course. Possibility is always possible.

Q: Hopefully and ideally, you would conduct a larger or at least additional similar studies to either confirm or dispute the findings in these studies, correct?

A: Ideally, yes.

Q: Now, let me ask you a question. In terms of randomization, if -- just to make sure I understand the concept, if I, for example, choose to vaccinate based solely on birth dates, would that be randomized?

A: Yes.

Q: And that would be considered a randomized study? A Yes.

(Exhibit Plaintiff-26 was marked for identification.)

BY MR. SIRI:

Q: I'm going hand you what's been marked, what is being marked as Plaintiff's Exhibit 24 -.26. Thank you. Sorry. This is the Peter Aaby study that you and I were talking about earlier, correct?

A: This is one of them.

Q: This is the study in which Peter Aaby found that children who receive DPT in the first six months of life versus those who got no vaccines died at ten times the rate, correct?

A: Right.

Q: And in this study, you earlier said that your concerns with Aaby's prior studies that had similar conclusions was that they weren't randomized; but in this study it was randomized, correct? Because it was -- strike that. In this study, in this study the vaccinated versus unvaccinated children were simply vaccinated or unvaccinated purely by the chance of when their birthday happened to be; isn't that correct?

A: Yes. It says they were allocated by birthday. I have to see. Well, you know, it's not absolutely clear as to how the randomization was done. Apparently there were periods of time when they were vaccinating and other periods when they were not vaccinating.

Q: I think that if you -- have you read this study before, Dr. Plotkin?

A: I've glanced at it, yes. I haven't read it thoroughly. But the, as I said before, the, this kind of study is useful. There's no doubt about that. But one needs to have some sort of immunological correlate to really confirm that that, that the findings are real. The other point is that Peter is working in an African community where there is a high mortality to begin with. And that's, of course, because of other factors. And so whether this would be true in, let's say, Denmark or elsewhere is not clear. And if my memory serves, attempts to show in Denmark what Peter has found in Africa have not been positive.

Q: Are you saying that there's a randomized study in Denmark comparing death rates between DPT and T -.

A: It was -.

Q: One second, Dr. Plotkin. Hold on. Hold on a second. I'm sorry. You've got to let me finish because the court reporter can't take down both of us talking. Okay? I'm asking is, is there a study from Denmark that compared children who received DTP versus children who received no vaccines at all that was randomized like this study was and that compared the death rate between the two groups?

A: Well, I'd have to go back and look, but my recollection is that because in Denmark everything is registered and they had excellent data on vaccines being given, that they did not find an effect on mortality of giving DTP. Regardless, my point is that mortality in the developed world is relatively rare in childhood; whereas, in Africa it's obviously common. Let me repeat what I said about Peter Aaby's work. It's not that I discard it or think that his conclusions are wrong. What I'm saying is that they are observational data, and they have to be confirmed by studies of the immune responses. And those have been done only to a certain degree.

Q: When you say "studies of immune response," what do you mean?

A: I mean, whether the immunity of the child is interfered with by DTP; that is, immunity to other diseases. And as I mentioned before, he had shown that measles has a positive, measles vaccine has a positive effect. And that has been confirmed by showing that measles vaccination influences immunity to other diseases.

Q: So what you're saying is you don't dispute his findings that at least in this African country -.

A: Yes.

Q: -- there is a ten-times-greater death rate amongst those who got DPT -- TP in the first six months of life versus those who got no vaccines, correct?

A: I don't dispute his findings. I would have to look further to make sure that the populations that were studied were absolutely equal in other respects.

Q: Okay.

A: But, again, I'm not one who discards Peter's studies a priori.

Q: Earlier you told me the issue was it wasn't randomized, but now -.

A: That is an important issue, yes.

Q: And it is, this one is randomized?

A: Well, again, I just have to be sure that it was randomized, that both groups were vaccinated or non-vaccinated at the same time rather than sequentially.

Q: Yes. Because it was done by birthdays. When people came into the clinics, right, depending on their birth date, they either got the vaccine or they didn't, correct? Correct?

A: Well, subject to my reading this carefully, I agree that he is claiming that it's randomized.

Q: So DTaP has been used around the world for what, 30, 40 years now, 50 years?

A: Mainly since the 1990s.

Q: Okay. Mainly since the 1990s.

A: So about 20 years.

Q: And Peter Aaby has been claiming, making this claim, a respected scientist whose conclusions you said you take seriously, that DTP might cause more deaths than people it saves -.

A: Yeah, I -.

Q: -- but -- let me just finish my question, please. When do you think this extra science on immunology you think is necessary is going to get done so we know whether or not DTP is saving more children than it kills?

A: Well, I would imagine that WHO is looking into it. I don't know that for a fact. But it also has to be pointed out that the vaccine that he's studying is whole-cell vaccine; it is not the vaccine being used in the United States.

Q: That's right. But it is being used in most third-world countries, correct?

A: In, the vaccines being used in the United States are being used in the U.S. and Europe.

Q: The DTP -.

A: But the DTP, the whole-cell vaccine is used very largely in Latin America and Africa.

Q: In developing countries?

A: Yes.

Q: Any reason that the life of a child in a developing country is not equal to that in the first-world country?

A: No.

Q: Okay.

A: But the whole-cell vaccine is considerably cheaper.

(Exhibit Plaintiff-27 was marked for identification.)

BY MR. SIRI:

Q: Dr. Plotkin, I'm going to hand you what's being marked as Plaintiff's Exhibit 24 -- 27. This is an excerpt from the 1994 IOM report, correct?

A: Yes.

Q: Under risk-modifying factors, the first sentence there says: The committee was able to identify little information pertaining to why some individuals react adversely to vaccines when most do not, correct?

A: Yes. Mm-hmm.

Q: Okay.

(Exhibit Plaintiff-28 was marked for identification.)

BY MR. SIRI:

Q: Handing you what's being marked as Plaintiff's Exhibit 28. I'm going to read you an excerpt from this, and I'm going to ask you a question. Okay, Dr. Plotkin?

A: Yes.

Q: Okay. It says: Both epidemiologic and mechanistic research suggests that most individuals who experience an adverse reaction to vaccines have a pre-existing susceptibility. These predispositions can exist for a number of reasons -.genetic variations in human or microbiome DNA, environmental exposures, behaviors, intervening illness, or developmental stage, to name just a few -- all of which can interact, as suggested graphically in figure 3-1. Some of these adverse reactions are specific to the particular vaccine, while others may not be. Some of these predispositions may be detectable to prior to the administration of vaccines. And then skipping down a little: Much work remains to be done to elucidate and develop strategies to document the immunologic mechanisms that lead to adverse effects in individual patients. Do you disagree with what the IOM wrote here?

A: Well, not in principle. If such factors can be identified. So far it has been very difficult to identify so-called predispositions.

Q: Is it not because, Dr. Plotkin, the science is just not being done to make those identified?

A: Some attempts have been made. There's a whole literature by Dr. Poland at the Mayo Clinic on such. But the things that he studied have been relatively minor reactions.

Q: Are you aware of any serious large-scale studies that have been done to assess the predispositions that might result in adverse reaction from a vaccine?

A: There have been some genetic studies done.

Q: By whom?

A: As I said, by the Mayo group in particular, and also some studies done Vanderbilt.

Q: Who did the studies Vanderbilt?

A: Well, James Crowe was one of the authors.

Q: What did the studies involve?

A: The studies involved looking at certain enzymes, particularly to see if there was an association with -- let's see. It was with -- I'm trying to remember which vaccine it was based on. Smallpox vaccine.

Q: Smallpox. Do people routinely get smallpox vaccine anymore in America?

A: No.

Q: Okay. Other than the researcher at Vanderbilt and the one at the Mayo Clinic that you mentioned, is there anybody else that you know of that is conducting any serious science to identify what might, what would render a child susceptible to a vaccine injury?

A: I think the people of British Columbia are doing some work.

Q: Who is that?

A: I can't remember the guy's name.

Q: Is it Chris Shaw?

A: Sorry?

Q: Is his name Chris Shaw?

A: Could be. It's a whole group of people at British Columbia.

Q: They've published good science in this area?

A: Yes.

Q: Respectable science?

A: Yes.

Q: And they are the ones who looked at aluminum adjuvants injected into lab animals in particular, correct?

A: They have done some work with aluminum adjuvants, yes.

Q: By showing that injecting aluminum can go to different parts of the animal, right?

A: Yes.

Q: I just want to make sure we're talking about the same group of scientists -.

A: Mm-hmm.

Q: -- at the University of British Columbia. Is, so do you recall if it's Chris Shaw and his group?

A: I don't recall specifically.

Q: Is -- okay. But it's the group at the University of British Columbia that's looking in particular at aluminum adjuvants in vaccines, correct, in animal models?

A: They're looking at a lot of different things, including adjuvants.

Q: Okay. Understood. And other than the group at British Columbia, Mayo Clinic, and Vanderbilt, are you aware of anybody else doing such science?

A: Not that I recall, no.

Q: Okay. If anybody would know, it'd be you, right, Dr. Plotkin?

A: Well, I don't read -- I cannot read every published scientific paper.

Q: Dr. Plotkin, I'm going to refer to the various forms of aluminum adjuvant used in vaccines as alum; is that okay?

A: Yes.

Q: Because there are different kinds, correct?

A: Yes.

Q: Okay. What is an antigen?

A: An antigen is usually a protein that induces an immune response.

Q: Antigens in killed vaccines, though, produce a very weak immune response, hence the need to add alum to the vaccine formulation, correct?

A: Frequently, not always.

Q: And alum, injected alum can increase the production of all kinds of cytokines, including IL-1, IL-2, IL-6, IL-17, correct?

A: Yes.

Q: Alum can be recovered from the injection site months or years after intramuscular injections, correct?

A: Well, it's, yeah, it's possible to find the alum. Of course, aluminum is a frequent, shall I say, present in all of us? We ingest a lot of it.

Q: I'm talking about injected aluminum. I'm asking, can it be recovered from the injection site months or years after intramuscular injection?

A: I believe it's possible, yes.

Q: In your book that you're holding in front of you, do you know if it says, quote: It is established that aluminum salt can be recovered at the injection site months or years after intramuscular injections?

A: Well, I'd have to look at it, but I don't doubt that that's, that could be in the book, yes.

Q: Okay. And antigen that is absorbed by alum can be taken up by macrophages and dendritic cells?

A: Yes.

Q: Macrophages is M-A-C-R-O-P-H-A-G-E-S. Macrophages are immune cells, correct?

A: Well, they are scavengers, basically.

Q: What do they do?

A: They take up antigens and present them to other cells.

Q: So that means that the alum as well as the antigen that's bound to it are taken up by macrophages and dendritic cells, correct?

A: Yes.

Q: Okay. Aluminum injected into the brain -.into the body can travel to the brain, correct?

A: I don't know that for a fact, but wouldn't be surprised.

Q: You've never seen any studies that show that aluminum injected into the body can travel to the brain?

A: I have not seen such studies, no, or not read such studies.

(Exhibit Plaintiff-29 was marked for identification.)

BY MR. SIRI:

Q: I'm going to hand you what's being marked as Plaintiff's Exhibit 29. Please take a look at that. In this study, do you have a problem with the journal that this study was published in?

A: No.

Q: Is the name of the journal Vaccine?

A: Yes.

Q: Are you a editor in that journal?

A: I was at one point.

Q: And you consider that to be a prestigious journal?

A: Yes.

Q: Okay. So in this study, conduct -- they found that injecting rabbits with aluminum and then dissected them, they found aluminum in the brain of the rabbits, correct?

A: Yes.

Q: Does that change your opinion of whether injecting aluminum can travel to the brain?

A: Well, it shows experimentally that that's the case. I'd have to look at the concentrations that were injected, whether they were reasonable with respect to what's injected into humans.

(Exhibit Plaintiff-30 was marked for identification.)

BY MR. SIRI:

Q: Here's another study. Here's another study that's being marked as Plaintiff's Exhibit 30. And this study involved mice. Can you please take a look at it. That study is from 2009, correct?

A: Yes.

MS. RUBY: Ms. Nieusma, did number 30 go through for you?MS. NIEUSMA: Yes. I'll let you know if I don't have anything .

BY MR. SIRI:

Q: And that study found that injecting aluminum in mice caused motor deficits and motor neuron degeneration, correct?

A: Apparently, yes. But, again, one has to compare the amounts injected with what's, what amounts are injected with vaccines.

Q: So in this study the authors note that they were attempting to use dose-equivalent amounts of alum vis-a-vis the vaccination schedule. I'll post that as a question, but I'll leave it to you to take -- you obviously, sounds like you never read this study, so you can take your time. Okay. Dr. Plotkin, there's no question pending about that study anymore. So let's move on.

A: Okay.

Q: Okay? So are you familiar with a study entitled "Delivery of Nanoparticles to Brain Metastases of Breast Cancer Using a Cellular Trojan Horse" from the Indiana University School of Medicine and Rice University?

A: No.

Q: Are you familiar with a study from 2013 entitled "Slow CCL2-dependent Translocation of Biopersistent Particles from Muscle to Brain"?

A: No.

Q: Are you familiar with the -- after this deposition, I'm happy to provide you copies of all these studies. You can take an opportunity to look at them. Are you familiar with a 2015 study entitled "Highly" -- actually, you know what? Before we continue, I'm going to mark this one. The study I just spoke about, I'm going to mark as Plaintiff's Exhibit 32.

(Exhibits Plaintiff-31 and Plaintiff-32 were marked for identification.)

BY MR. SIRI:

Q: I'm going hand this to you. In this study, if you turn to page 5, you can actually see pictures of the brain of dissected mice injected with aluminum and pictures of the aluminum in the brain. Let me know when you've had an opportunity to look at that.

A: Yes. Okay.

(Exhibit Plaintiff-33 was marked for identification.)

BY MR. SIRI:

Q: Okay. That's from 2013. I'm going to show you another study from 2015 being marked Plaintiff's Exhibit No. 33. This study involved 155 mice, again injected with aluminum. And, again, you can find pictures of the aluminum in the dissected mice in their brains. Since we're running short on time, I won't hand you all the studies on this. But having had an opportunity just for the last few minutes to look at a few of these studies, do you have any -.can aluminum injected into the body travel to the brain?

A: Well, there are experiments suggesting that that is possible.

Q: Okay.

A: The, in particular, there's a, I know there's a French group that's been, let's say, working on the potential dangers of aluminum as well as the British Columbia group. What we lack is evidence in humans that such phenomena are causing the problems that are being caused in mice, and that may relate to dose issues.

Q: Isn't that because those studies would be unethical, Dr. Plotkin?

A: No, I wouldn't say they'd be unethical. I would say that looking for aluminum deposits in the brains of people at autopsy, et cetera, that's entirely feasible.

Q: And so if they did autopsies of people's brains and they found aluminum, then that would be a cause for concern?

A: It could be. But one would need to combine that or look at the symptoms of the patients whose brains are being examined.

(Exhibit Plaintiff-34 was marked for identification.)

BY MR. SIRI:

Q: I'm going to hand you one final study on this. It's been marked Plaintiff's Exhibit 34. This one they were very careful, my understanding is, to do a number of different doses to see the response.

A: This is the French group.

Q: That study is the French group, right, that I think you were referring to earlier?

A: Yes.

Q: Okay. So in any event, if aluminum bound to antigen does travel to the brain, Dr. Plotkin, and remains there, would that cause an immune activation event in the brain?

A: I don't know whether it would or not. I'm not -.

Q: Do you think it could result in neurodevelopmental disorders?

A: Again, there's no evidence that that's the case.

(Exhibit Plaintiff-35 was marked for identification.)

BY MR. SIRI:
Q: I'm going to hand you what's being marked -- I'm going to hand you what's marked Exhibit 35. Are you familiar with -- are you familiar with this book?
A: No.
Q: Well, then I'll give you a copy today when you leave.
MS. RUBY: Okay. Ms. Nieusma, Exhibit 35 is uploading, but it might take just one second.
MS. NIEUSMA: Okay. No problem .
BY MR. SIRI:
Q: Dr. Plotkin, has an increase in IL-6 been shown to induce autism-like features in lab animals?
A: Well, IL-6 is an inflammatory cytokine. And its relationship to autism, I would say, is not clear. But it is an important cytokine.
Q: Has it been shown to induce autism-like features in animals when injected into animals for experimentation?
A: I'm not aware of that, but it's quite possible that that could happen if you use enough IL-6.
Q: Do you know the maximum amount -- strike that. Are you familiar with the study out of -- are you familiar with the study entitled "Inhibition of IL-6 Trans-Signaling in the Brain Increases Social Ability in the BTBR Mouse Model of Autism"?
A: No.
Q: Are you familiar with the study called "Maternal Immune Activation Alters Fetal Brain Development through Interleukin-6"?
A: Vaguely, yes. Yeah.
Q: Published in the Journal of Neuroscience?
A: Yeah, well, I don't remember the journal.
Q: Is that one of the journals you consider respectable?
A: Yes.
Q: And this was out of the University of California Medical Center. This is from California Institute, CalTech. That institution did a number of studies regarding -- that group did a number of studies relating to immune activation and neurological disorder, correct?
A: Yes.
Q: And they found a connection between immune activation and neurological historical disorders, correct?
A: Mm-hmm.
Q: And one of the -- is that a yes?
A: Yes.
Q: Okay. And one of the study's findings they had was that immune activation alters fetal brain development through interleukin-6, correct?
A: As I said before, IL-6 is an important cytokine. I would point out in relation to immune activation, that immune activation occurs as a result of disease and exposure to a variety of stimuli, not just vaccines.
Q: But it can be caused by vaccines, correct?
A: Immune activation is the objective of vaccines.
Q: Do you know the maximum amount of the aluminum that is injected into a child who follows the CDC schedule?

A: I haven't done the arithmetic, but I believe it would amount to several milligrams.

(Exhibit Plaintiff-36 was marked for identification.)

BY MR. SIRI:
Q: I'm going hand you what's been marked as Plaintiff's Exhibit 36. Okay? And before I do that, question for you: The group out of the British Columbia that you were -- the group out of the University of British Columbia, that's out of the Department of Ophthalmology and Visual Sciences?
A: Yeah.
Q: I'm going to hand you a letter from, what's been marked as Exhibit 36, which is a letter from one of the professors that runs the lab in that group?
VIDEO OPERATOR: We have four minutes left on the disc.
MR. SIRI: Okay .
BY MR. SIRI:
Q: Have you seen this letter before?
A: No.
Q: Okay. This letter is from the group at the University of British Columbia you mentioned before, correct?
A: Yes.
Q: And it's addressed to HHS, correct?
A: Yes.
Q: As well as NIH?
A: Yes.
Q: FDA and CDC, correct?
A: Yes.
Q: Okay. In the first paragraph, can you read the first paragraph?
A: I am writing to you in regard to aluminum adjuvants in vaccines. The subject is one my laboratory works on intensively and, therefore, where I feel I have some expertise. In particular, we have studied the impact of aluminum adjuvants in animal models of neurological disease, including autism spectrum disorder. Our relevant studies on the general topic of aluminum neurotoxicity in general and specifically in regard to adjuvants are cited below.
Q: Now, can you read the last sentence in the next paragraph.
A: In children there is growing evidence that aluminum adjuvants may disrupt developmental processes in the central nervous system and, therefore, contribute to ASD in susceptible children.
Q: And just the next paragraph.
A: Despite the foregoing, the safety of aluminum adjuvants in vaccines has not been properly studied in humans, even though pursuant to the recommended vaccine schedule published by the Centers for Disease Control, a baby may be injected with up to 3.675 micrograms of aluminum adjuvants by six months of age.
Q: Just the next sentence and I guess we can wrap up.
A: And in regards to the above, it is my belief that the CDC's claim on its website that vaccines do not cause autism is wholly unsupported. So my comments are, one, that my estimate was pretty much correct. Second, that, unfortunately, Dr. Shaw has been associated with the party that I mentioned before, Tomljenovic, who, in my view, is completely

untrustworthy as far as scientific data are concerned. So I'm concerned about Dr. Shaw being influenced by that individual. And the, I'm not aware that there is evidence that aluminum disrupts the developmental processes in susceptible children.

Q: Dr. Shaw is a scientist that studies aluminum regularly, correct?

A: Yes.

Q: Do you study aluminum regularly?

A: No.

MR. SIRI: Okay. Are we done?

VIDEO OPERATOR: Yep. This ends tape four of the deposition of Dr. Stanley Plotkin. We are going off the record. The time is 16:33.

(Brief recess.)

Part 5

VIDEO OPERATOR: This is the beginning of Disc No. 5, the deposition of Dr. Stanley Plotkin. We are on the record. The time is 16:43.

BY MR. SIRI:

Q: Now, Dr. Plotkin, I'm handing you what has been marked as Plaintiff's Exhibits 37 and 38.

(Exhibits Plaintiff-37 and Plaintiff-38 were marked for identification.)

BY MR. SIRI:

Q: Are these letters also written by individuals who are very experienced in studying aluminum adjuvant?

A: Yes. Well, one of the letters -.

Q: Okay.

A: -- is from a French group. And I would point out that -.

MS. NIEUSMA: Remember, just yes or no answers, Dr. Plotkin. We're trying to get you out of here -- out of there.

THE WITNESS: Yes .

BY MR. SIRI:

Q: Okay. And is the content of these letters similar to that of the letter from Chris Shaw?

A: Yes.

(Exhibit Plaintiff-39 was marked for identification.)

BY MR. SIRI:

Q: Dr. Plotkin, I'm going to hand you what's been marked as Plaintiff's Exhibit 39. Okay. This is a study entitled "Aluminum in the Brain Tissue in Autism," correct?

A: Yes.

Q: And it was published in the Journal of Trace Elements in Medicine and Biology, correct?

A: Yes.

Q: And it found, and according to its author, he found what he says is some of the highest values of aluminum in human tissue yet recorded in the brains of these autistic children who died prematurely, correct?

A: Well, I'd have to read the paper, but apparently that's the case.

Q: And do you know that the stand-out observation in this study is that the aluminum that he found was in the immune cells of the brain, including within immune cells traveling into the brain?

A: Yes. But they were not associated with neurons.

Q: They also found aluminum in the neurons as well, Dr. Plotkin, correct?

A: But mostly in other cells.

Q: And immune-related cells, right, immune-system-related cells?

A: Cells that travel, yes.

Q: What is encephalitis?

A: Inflammation of the brain.

Q: What is encephalopathy?

A: Well, it's a vague term that means something's wrong with the brain.

Q: What is encephalomyelitis?

A: Inflammation of the brain.

Q: Do all five of the DTaP-containing vaccines sold in this country list encephalopathy within seven days of a prior pertussis-containing vaccine as a contraindication?

A: In other words, if encephalitis is present at the time of vaccination?

Q: Mm-hmm.

A: Yes, I imagine so.

Q: No. Meaning that if there was encephalopathy within seven days of a prior pertussis-containing vaccination, that's a contraindication to getting more pertussis vaccination?

A: Oh, yes.

Q: Okay. And do all three of the hepatitis A-containing vaccines sold in this country list encephalitis or encephalopathy as a reported adverse reaction in Section 6.2 of their product inserts?

A: Well, I don't know that for sure, but I imagine that it is a contraindication.

Q: Do all three of the hepatitis B-containing vaccines sold in this country list either encephalitis or encephalopathy as a reported adverse reaction in Section 6.2 of their product insert?

A: Yes.

Q: Do almost all of the flu vaccines sold in this country list encephalopathy or encephalomyelitis as a reported adverse reaction in 6.2 -.

A: Yes.

Q: -- of their insert? Does the only chicken pox vaccine sold in this country list encephalitis as a reported adverse reaction?

A: Yes.

Q: Why do you think brain swelling after vaccination is being reported in all of these vaccines?

A: Anything that happens after vaccination is included in contraindications. That they are related causally is not necessarily the case.

Q: What is the total quantity of antigen in most pediatric vaccines?

A: Well, that's vary variable. I mean, perhaps up to 50 milligrams. Depends entirely on the vaccine.

Q: Miniscule amount, though, very tiny?

A: Yes.

Q: Almost -- could you even see it with the naked eye if you had it?

A: Yeah, you could in some cases, yes.

Q: Some cases?

A: Mm-hmm.

Q: But for most vaccines, it would probably be very difficult?

A: Yes.

Q: Okay. Are there any ingredients in vaccines that you're aware of that can damage neurons?

A: Not that I'm aware of, no.

Q: Are there any vaccines, any ingredients in vaccines that you're aware of that can damage human cells?

A: Oh, well, I mean, that depends on the concentrations and so forth. Human cells, of course, are susceptible to lots of substances. But, again, it's very much dependent on the concentration.

Q: Do any of the vaccines on the childhood schedule contain monkey kidney cells?

A: Well, the polio vaccine does.

Q: Okay. Go ahead. I'm sorry.

A: Go ahead. I'll stop there.

Q: Are the monkey kidneys used in making the polio vaccine removed from the monkey while the animal is still alive?

A: These days much of the polio vaccine is produced in a continuous cell line of, derived from monkeys rather than from monkeys, from live monkeys, so to speak. So I'm pretty sure that the IPOL vaccine, for example, is produced in vero cells.

Q: Okay. And when you say "continuous cell line," what do you mean by that?

A: I mean a cell that grows continuously derived from tissues that were normal tissues to begin with.

Q: I'm sorry. Say that again, Doctor.

A: So they are cells that continue to multiply, unlike cells from a, let's say, from a kidney that will not continuously multiply. These are cells derived from the kidney that will continue to multiply and, therefore, can be used to make vaccines in.

Q: Cells that continue to multiply unabated are typically considered cancerous, right?

A: Well, if, depends on the circumstances in the cells. But it's true that cancer cells do continue to replicate indefinitely. The vero cells are only used at certain passage levels. They're not used, you know, a thousand passages further on.

Q: In relation to the amount of polio antigen in the final polio vaccine product, how much monkey kidney cell material is there in the final product? Is it about the same amount? Is there more monkey kidney cell? Is there less?

A: No. I can't give you a figure offhand. But the, I am pretty sure that the amount of polio antigen is superior to the amount of kidney antigen.

Q: But you're not sure?

A: I don't recall the exact amounts.

Q: Monkey cellular material remaining in the vaccine is considered either impurities or byproduct of the manufacturing process, correct?

A: Yes.

Q: Do any vaccines in the childhood vaccine schedule contain blood serum from calves or other bovines?

A: Well, frequently calf serum is used to make the vaccine, but calf serum is removed before the vaccine is used because you don't want to sensitize the vaccinee to cows.

Q: Meaning if there was cow serum remaining in the vaccine, the child could develop antibodies to essentially cow -.

A: Yes.

Q: -- cow products?

A: Yes.

Q: And that would be -- and they could develop an allergy to it, right?

A: If there were, yes.

Q: If there were calf serum in the vaccines, correct?

A: Yes.

Q: But you're saying there's no calf serum in vaccines, right?

A: It is removed, yes.

(Exhibit Plaintiff-40 was marked for identification.)

BY MR. SIRI:

Q: Dr. Plotkin, I'm going to hand you what's been marked as Plaintiff's Exhibit 40. What is this?

A: Vaccine Excipient & Media Summary.

Q: And who produces this document, the CDC, correct, or the FDA?

A: I think it's the FDA.

Q: Okay. And this lists the ingredients contained in various vaccines, correct?

A: Yes.

Q: Can you go to Kinrix on the first page. That's K-I-N-R-I-X.

A: Yes.

Q: DTaP-IPV. Do you see in the third line down it says: Calf serum?

A: Yeah. Well, that is used to grow the polio virus.

Q: Right. And this is one of the ingredients that remains in the vaccine?

A: I do not believe so. I mean, the vaccine, as I said, is made using calf serum as a nutrient, but it is then -.

Q: Removed because, otherwise, it would be dangerous, you said, right?

A: Yes. Yes.

Q: Can you go to the top of this document. You see it says -- you know what? Let me ask you a few other questions, and then we'll come back to this document, Dr. Plotkin. Few quick questions and then we'll come back to it. Do any vaccines on the childhood schedule contain embryonic guinea pig cultures?

A: Embryonic guinea pig. I don't think any current vaccine is made in guinea pig cells. Varicella vaccine was passaged in guinea pig cells, but certainly not made in guinea pig cells.

Q: Do you know if any vaccines contain cows' milk in it or products from cow -.

A: Cows' what?

Q: Any product derived from cows' milk, any component derived from cows' milk?

A: Oh, well, could be, casein, for example, could be -.

Q: Casein -.

A: -- could be used.

Q: Dr. Plotkin -- Dr. Plotkin, and if there was casein in the vaccine, a child could become sensitized to that, correct?

A: No, I'm not sure about that.

Q: You're not sure anymore about that?

A: No.

Q: Yeah.

A: I think there are other sensitizing things in calf serum.

Q: Dr. Plotkin, can I see that a second. Did I give you the right one? So earlier you said -- okay. So do any vaccines contain egg protein?

A: Oh, yes. Influenza vaccines.

Q: And do those remain in the final product?

A: I believe they do, yes. Not huge amounts, but there are traces certainly.

Q: Do any vaccines contain gelatin from pigs?

A: Yes.

Q: Do any vaccines contain gelatin from cows?

A: Actually, I think in Muslim countries, they have tried to do that. But mostly it's from pig.

Q: Do any vaccines contain recombinant GMO yeast?

A: Recombinant GMOs. Yes, I imagine so, yes.

Q: Are there any other animal products, parts, cells, material, or any other kind that you are aware of that are contained in any vaccine in the pediatric schedule?

A: Well, aside from trace amounts, no.

MS. NIEUSMA: Guys, unfortunately, my 5:00 is here, so I've got to cut this short.

MR. SIRI: Well, we're not, we're not done. So we need to, you know, so we're going to -.

BY MR. SIRI:

Q: Can you come back tomorrow morning, Dr. Plotkin?

A: No. Absolutely not.

MR. SIRI: Okay. Well, Counsel, we need to, how long is your -- you need to move whatever you have right now, then.

MS. NIEUSMA: No, I don't.

MR. SIRI: I'm not done with the deposition.

MS. NIEUSMA: Then re-notice it for A second day.

MR. SIRI: I don't -- no. The notice says: From day to day. He's under subpoena. He needs to be here today. It's only, it's only 5:00. And it says: From day to day. So tomorrow's the next day.

MS. NIEUSMA: If he's not available, he's not available. You guys can feel free to have him held in contempt while he's in Pennsylvania, but I gotta go.

MS. RUBY: Are you available in a half an hour or something, that we could take a short break?

MS. NIEUSMA: Yeah, I can do that.

MR. SIRI: Okay. So let us know when you're done. Half an hour. We'll start at 5:30, then, or if you get done earlier.

THE WITNESS: Does she have to be present?

MR. SIRI: Do you mind if we continue without you being present? Dr. Plotkin says he's fine with continuing without you.

MS. NIEUSMA: As long as he's okay with that, that's fine with me. I think he's got a pretty good handle on things. So I'm not too concerned.

MR. SIRI: Okay. Great. Then we'll continue.

MS. NIEUSMA: All right.

106

MR. SIRI: Thank you.

MS. RUBY: Ms. Nieusma, if you want to rejoin the conversation, obviously you can dial back in.

MS. NIEUSMA: Yeah. I'm just going to leave you guys on speaker in my office and do this in the conference room and I'll be back.

MS. RUBY: Okay .

BY MR. SIRI:

Q: Do any vaccines on the childhood vaccine schedule contain MRC-5 human diploid cells?

A: Yes.

Q: What are these?

A: Rubella, varicella, hepatitis A.

Q: What are MRC-5 cells?

A: They are human fibroblast cell strain.

Q: And how are they created?

A: They were created by taking fetal tissue and, from a particular fetus that was aborted by maternal choice. And the cells, so-called fibroblast cells were cultivated from that tissue. The fibroblast cells replicate for about 50 passages and then die.

Q: So MRC-5 cells are cultured cell lines from aborted fetal tissue?

A: They're not cell lines.

Q: What are they?

A: They're cell strains cultivated from an aborted fetus, yes.

Q: So cell strains from an aborted fetus?

A: Yes. Yeah. They're not immortal.

Q: They live for five generations and then they die?

A: About 50 generations.

Q: About 50 generations and then they die?

A: Yes.

Q: And then how is more MRC-5 created?

A: Well, a seed stock is made of early passage cells so that one can go back to the seed stock, which is, let's say, at the, more or less the eighth passage and make new cells at the 20th passage and use those to make the vaccine.

Q: Okay. So these are, these cell strains are human cells?

A: Yes.

Q: Do any vaccines on the childhood vaccine schedule contain WI-38 human diploid lung fibroblast?

A: Well, they used to, but I don't think anything is made in those cells anymore. They have been replaced by MRC-5.

Q: So you're not aware of any vaccine that has in its final formulation WI-38 human diploid lung fibroblasts?

A: As I said, at one point in the past, RA 27/3, for example, rubella vaccine, was grown in WI-38. But the supply is insufficient, so MRC-5 is now used.

Q: And these, and WI-38 was created from an aborted fetus?

A: Yes.

Q: fetus? They took the lung tissue from the aborted

A: Yes.

Q: correct? And f rom that they'd grown this cell line,

A: Yes. Cell strain.

Q: Cell strain. Is this cell line immortal?

A: No.

Q: Do any vaccines in the childhood vaccine schedule contain human albumin?

A: Oh, yes.

Q: What is human albumin?

A: Human albumin is part of human serum.

Q: And what is human serum?

A: What is human serum? Human serum is part of the blood that is liquid.

Q: Right. It's the non-red blood cell part of the -.

A: Yes.

Q: -- of the blood, right? From where was it obtained?

A: The human serum?

Q: Yes.

A: Well, that would be variable from donors who are healthy donors. That's all I can say to that.

Q: How is it used in the manufacturing process?

A: I'm sorry?

Q: How is it used in the manufacturing process?

A: Well, serum is used to keep cells healthy during the process of making a vaccine. So, in other words, since the vaccines or some vaccines have to be grown in cells, you have to keep the cells in a good state.

Q: So the cells that are used -- the virus or bacteria -- the viruses used in some of the vaccines are grown in this human blood component?

A: Well, yes. I believe that the serum is removed in the final product, but certainly it's important to keep the cells healthy during the manufacture of the vaccine.

Q: Do you think that -- so none of it remains in the final product?

A: I don't believe so, no.

Q: Because that could be problematic, right?

A: Well, it could be. I mean, if the individual is not, not healthy.

Q: Right. Or if maybe some of the, you know, human blood components bind to some of the aluminum and develop antibodies, self-antibodies, correct?

A: If they develop antibodies against the serum component, that would not be good.

Q: Right. What, do any vaccines contain human material in them that -- I'm sorry. Strike that. Apologies. Do any vaccines in the childhood vaccine schedule contain recombinant human albumin?

A: Yes.

Q: What is recombinant human albumin, A-L-B-U-M-I-N?

A: So it's a component of human serum which is useful to stabilize cells and keep them healthy, and it's made by genetic engineering.

Q: Okay. So it's genetically engineered human serum basically?

A: Part of human serum, yes.

Q: Is that, are these genetically engineered protein structures?

A: Yes. And the idea was to eliminate any possibility of a contaminant from human albumin obtained from the donors. So it's made in cells, using the DNA for albumin, and that way one can be sure that there's no contaminant.

Q: And, again, you pretty much want to make sure that none of that remained in the final product, too, right?

A: Well, human albumin is probably not much of a problem in terms of causing reactions. So -.

Q: But in terms of it potentially binding to the alum, that could be problematic, correct?

A: Well, I don't know the answer to that question.

Q: Okay. The vaccines that contain human material in them, they also contain human DNA and protein, correct?

A: They may, yes.

Q: Isn't it true that human DNA in vaccines is typically purposefully fragmented to below 500 base pairs in length?

A: Yes. One doesn't, you know, I would say mostly for theoretical reasons, doesn't want to put DNA into, attacked DNA into vaccines. I think the actual risk is zero, but that's my opinion.

Q: Isn't it true that MMR II contains approximately 150 nanograms cells substrate double-strand DNA and single-strand DNA per dose purposefully fragmented to approximately 215 baste base pairs in length?

A: Yeah, that's probably correct, yes.

Q: And is it true that VARIVAX, vaccine for chicken pox, is manufactured using WI-38 and MRC-5 -.

A: Yes.

Q: -- and contains approximately two micrograms of cell substrate double-strand DNA or approximately 1 trillion fragments of human DNA?

A: It may be true.

Q: Isn't it true that the Havrix, the hepatitis A vaccine, also contains millions of fragments of human DNA?

A: Likely.

Q: Do you know whether strands of DNA below 500 base pairs are now known to insert themselves into living cells with which they come into contact?

A: I do not have that information, but the likelihood that they would be genetically included in the genome of vaccinees, in my view, is zero.

Q: Do you have a study to support that view?

A: I do not have a study that supports that view. But it is, to me, unlikely that the DNA would travel from the site of injection to the semen or the ovaries.

Q: Could it insert into itself DNA even in the muscle tissue or if it gets into the blood into -.

A: Theoretically. But that's not going to mean that it's going to have any impact on the individual.

Q: Are you familiar with the insertional mutagenesis?

A: Yes.

Q: Do you have any study to show that injecting millions of pieces of human DNA into babies and children is safe?

A: The only studies are all the safety studies that have been done on vaccines.

Q: And you can produce those studies, right?

A: Well, those studies are available from the manufacturers and from CDC, and I'm not aware of any data showing that the inheritable characteristic was transmitted by a vaccine.

Q: So you don't, you don't personally don't know of any study that shows the safety of injecting human, millions pieces of human DNA into babies?

A: Such studies are general safety studies, and I haven't yet seen the vaccinee develop a new genetic trait as a result of vaccination.

Q: Is it possible it can cause cancer?

A: Anything is possible, but there are no data to support that.

Q: Is there data to show that it doesn't do that?

A: Yes. Observations made over millions of vaccinees.

Q: Okay. And you have the studies to show that, right?

A: The studies are easily available in terms of vaccine safety studies that have been done by many, many people.

Q: Excellent. Then it should be very easy for you to direct me to those and can provide copies?

A: Yes.

Q: Wonderful.

A: You can read the chapter on vaccine safety.

Q: Vaccines contain dead or weakened polio virus, correct?

A: IPV does, yes.

Q: Beginning in the 1950s, polio vaccines were routinely grown on nonhuman primate kidney cells, correct?

A: Correct.

Q: Are you aware of any simian monkey viruses, meaning viruses that come from primates, that contaminated polio vaccines and infected individuals receiving the polio vaccine?

A: Yes. SV40.

Q: What does that SV40 stand for?

A: Simian virus 40.

Q: Was it the 40th simian virus found?

A: Yes.

Q: Are you aware of any other simian viruses that are in any vaccine?

A: At this stage, no.

Q: Are you aware of any bovine virus that is in any vaccine?

A: Well, bovine virus. Nothing comes to mind at the moment.

Q: Are you aware of any virus from any animal other than simian or bovine that is in any vaccine?

A: Yes. There's a pig virus present in one of the rotavirus vaccines.

Q: What is that virus called?

A: Circovirus.

Q: Is there more than one type, or is there only one?

A: There's more than one type, but I think only one was recovered from the vaccine.

Q: Which one is that?

A: I think it was 2.

Q: Circovirus 2.

A: I think so.

Q: Are you aware of any retrovirus that are in any vaccine?

A: Retroviruses? No.

Q: Are you aware of any prions that are in any vaccine?

A: No.

Q: Are you aware of any human viruses that are in any vaccine apart from the virus for which the vaccine is intended?

A: No.

Q: You indicated that they did find a porcine circovirus type 2 in rotavirus, correct?

A: Yes.

Q: Was that unintentional?

A: Yes.

Q: When it was released to the market, they didn't know that virus was in there, correct?

A: Correct.

Q: And when they released the polio vaccine on the market, they didn't know SV40 was in there, correct?

A: Correct.

Q: Are you aware of how many micrograms of 2-phen, P-H-E-N-O-X-Y-E-T-H-A-N-O-L? How do you pronounce that?

A: 2-phenoxyethanol.

Q: Yeah. Are you aware of how many micrograms of 2-phenoxyethanol a child following the childhood vaccine schedule would be injected with?

A: No. I'd have to look that up.

Q: Do you think it's close to around a hundred micrograms?

A: It could be, but I'd have to look it up.

Q: Do you know safe level in terms of that ingredient?

A: I am not aware that there, that there is toxicity associated with 2-phenoxyethanol. It's a fairly harmless substance, as far as I'm aware.

Q: Do you know any vaccines in the childhood schedule that include ferric nitrate?

A: Ferric nitrate? No, I don't recall that.

Q: Are you aware of how many micrograms of polysorbate 80 a child following the vaccine schedule would be injected with?

A: I don't have the amount, no.

Q: Now, I'm going to give you back Exhibit 40, Dr. Plotkin. Take a look at that a moment. You indicated that you weren't aware that WI-38 was in the final vaccine product. If you could turn to page 3 for MMR and MMR V.

A: (Witness complies.)

Q: Do you see that within the ingredient list that lists WI-38 human diploid lung fibroblast?

A: Yes, I do see that.

Q: I believe that of the ingredients that we discussed until now, the rest of them you indicated you are aware are in vaccines except for -- are there any ingredients we discussed until now that you believe are not in vaccines?

A: Well, I'd have to go back over all the questions you asked, but I do want to say that WI-38, as I said before, was the original fibroblast cell line. And I think that manufacturers have significantly shifted to MRC-5. But WI-38 could still be used. I don't see anything wrong with that.

Q: Are there any vaccine ingredients that are not listed on the FDA's official vaccine excipient and media summary table that you're aware of?

A: I don't see how I can really answer that question without reading the whole thing. But I imagine that it's a complete list.

Q: Okay. Isn't it true that an adjuvant will bind not only to the target antigen but also to the impurities and byproduct of the manufacturing process?

A: Probably, yes.

Q: And those impurities and byproducts are all listed in what has been marked as Exhibit No. 40, correct?

A: Yes.

Q: Okay. Once the impurities or byproducts are bound to the aluminum, the body may also develop antibodies to these impurities and byproducts, correct?

A: "May" is the operative word, but not necessarily.

Q: The entire purpose of the aluminum binding to a protein structure, be it an antigen or some other protein structure, is to cause an immune response that would develop antibodies, correct?

A: Yes. But the protein has to be of the right size and presentation in order to induce an immune response. And that will not always be the case if the protein is small or is something not recognize by the human immune system.

Q: Do you know whether the protein structure for any of the ingredients on Exhibit 40 are not the right size to bind to alum?

A: Well, I think it's unlikely. The monosodium glutamate, for example, will cause an immune response. I have to look through the whole thing. Amino acids probably are unlikely to induce an immune response.

Q: Anything else?

A: You want me to read this whole thing?

Q: Oh, no. I'm just asking, in terms of just the stuff that's got protein structures in it.

A: Well, things like calf serum, if they were present, would, would possibly induce an immune response. But the things on this list, the vast majority of them are unlikely to do so.

Q: Because they're not protein structures?

A: They're not proteins or they're very small.

Q: Okay. Other than the -- strike that. How about, and we talked earlier, human albumin, that would be of a big enough protein structure to bind to alum, correct?

A: It could, although the fact that it's human means that individuals might well not respond to -- that is, not respond to human albumin as a foreign protein.

Q: Right. Maybe not alone, right? But bound to alum it might, correct?

A: It might. But I'm not aware of evidence that it does.

Q: Are you aware of a study that looked at that issue?

A: I have not read such a study, no.

Q: How about the human DNA, do you believe that the human DNA strands can bind to the alum?

A: No.

Q: Why is that?

A: I don't see any chemical reason why it should.

Q: Any reason why it shouldn't?

A: Proving a negative is always more difficult.

Q: Well, I'm just trying to know if you know or you're just, you're not sure. That's all. I'm not asking -- I'm just saying if you don't know, just say you don't know. That's fine.

A: I have no reason to believe that DNA will bind to albumin.

Q: But you don't know for sure?

A: I have not done the experiment, no.

Q: Okay. And do you know whether it will bind to any of the cellular debris from MRC-5 or WI-38?

A: Whether human albumin would bind?

Q: No. Whether alum would bind to MRC-5 or any of the cellular debris that's in the final product from MRC-5 or -.

A: Oh, I think it could, but I don't know that it does.

Q: Do you know whether alum could bind to any of the cellular debris from WI-38?

A: It might, but I don't know that for a fact.

Q: Do you know whether alum would bind to any of the gelatin from pigs?

A: I think that's unlikely.

Q: Why is that?

A: I don't think that alum would bind to gelatin, but I don't know that for a fact.

Q: What about egg protein; could alum bind to egg protein?

A: Possibly.

Q: And to casein?

A: I suppose it's possible, but I'm not aware of any evidence.

Q: You don't know?

A: I don't know.

Q: Okay. In your work related to vaccines, how many fetuses have been part of that work?

A: My own personal work? Two.

Q: Two. So in your, in all of your work related to vaccines throughout your whole career, you've only ever worked with two fetuses?

A: In terms of making vaccines, yes. Yes.

(Exhibit Plaintiff-41 was marked for identification.)

BY MR. SIRI:

Q: I'm going to hand you, I'm going to hand you what's been marked Plaintiff's Exhibit 41. Okay? Are you familiar with this article, Dr. Plotkin?

A: Yes.

Q: Are you listed as an author on this article?

A: Yes.

Q: This study took place at the Wistar Institute, correct?

A: Yes.

Q: You were at the Wistar Institute, correct?

A: Yes.

Q: How many fetuses were used in the study described in this article?

A: Quite a few. But my answer to the previous question was what did I use to make vaccines, and the answer was two.

Q: Can you read back the question I had asked.COURT REPORTER: Just now or prior?

MR. SIRI: No. Prior. - - .

(Whereupon, the Reporter read back a preceding portion of the testimony as directed: "Q. In your work related to vaccines, how many fetuses have been part of that work? "A. My own personal work? Two.")

BY MR. SIRI:

Q: So I'm going to ask that question again. In your work related to vaccines, how many fetuses were involved in that work?

A: There were only two fetuses involved in making vaccines. When fetal strains of, fibroblast strains were first developed, I was involved in that work trying to characterize those cells; but they were not used to make vaccines.

Q: Wasn't the purpose of this study to help develop a human cell line or to support the use of human cell lines in the creation of vaccines?

A: The idea was to study the cell strains from fetuses to determine whether or not they could be used to make vaccines.

Q: So this was related to your work?

A: Well, yes, in a sense -.

Q: To vaccines, correct?

A: Yes. It was preparatory.

Q: So this study involved 74 fetuses, correct?

A: I don't remember exactly how many.

Q: If you turn to page 12 of the study.

A: Seventy-six.

Q: Seventy-six. And these fetuses were all three months or older when aborted, correct?

A: Yes.

Q: And these were all normally developed fetuses, correct?

A: Yes.

Q: Okay. These included fetuses that were aborted for social and psychiatric reasons, correct?

A: Correct.

Q: What organs did you harvest from these fetuses?

A: Well, I didn't personally harvest any, but a whole range of tissues were harvested by co-workers.

Q: And these pieces were then cut up into little pieces, right?

A: Yes.

Q: And they were cultured?

A: Yes.

Q: Some of the pieces of the fetuses were pituitary gland that were chopped up into pieces to -.

A: Mm-hmm.

Q: Included the lung of the fetuses?

A: Yes.

Q: Included the skin?

A: Yes.

Q: Kidney?

A: Yes.

Q: Spleen?

A: Yes.

Q: Heart?

A: Yes.

Q: Tongue?

A: I don't recall, but probably yes.

Q: So I just want to make sure I understand. In your entire career -- this was just one study. So I'm going to ask you again, in your entire career, how many fetuses have you worked with approximately?

A: Well, I don't remember the exact number, but quite a few when we were studying them originally before we decided to use them to make vaccines.

Q: Do you have any sense? I mean, this one study had 76. How many other studies did you have that you used aborted fetuses for?

A: I don't remember how many.

Q: You're aware, are you aware that the, one of the objections to vaccination by the plaintiff in this case is the inclusion of aborted fetal tissue in the development of vaccines and the fact that it's actually part of the ingredients of vaccines?

A: Yeah, I'm aware of those objections. The Catholic church has actually issued a document on that which says that individuals who need the vaccine should receive the vaccines, regardless of the fact, and that I think it implies that I am the individual who will go to hell because of the use of aborted tissues, which I am glad to do.

Q: Do you know if the mother's Catholic?

A: I have no idea.

Q: Okay.

A: But she should consult her priest.

Q: If she has a -- if she's, in fact, Christian, I guess, right? In any event, so we have 76 in this study. Would you approximate it's been a few hundred fetuses?

A: Oh, no, I don't think it was that many. Probably not many more than in this paper. And I should stipulate that we had nothing to do with the cause of the abortion.

Q: Some of these were for psychiatric institutions, correct?

A: Actually, all I can say is that the fetuses that I personally worked with actually came from Sweden, from a Swedish co-worker. And so I, in no case, was able to determine what exactly the reason for the abortion was.

Q: I'm just asking you, some of the fetuses that you did use did come from abortions from people who were in psychiatric institutions, correct?

A: I don't know that. What I'm telling you is that I got them from a co-worker; and if it's stated in the paper, it's true. But, otherwise, I do not know.

Q: So if it's in the paper, you don't contest it, right?

A: I don't contest it, no.

Q: Okay. Have you ever used orphans to study an experimental vaccine?

A: Yes.

Q: Have you ever used the mentally handicapped to study an experimental vaccine?

A: I don't recollect ever doing studies in mentally handicapped individuals. At the time in the 1960s, it was not an uncommon practice.

Q: So you're saying -- I'm not clear on your answer. I'm sorry. Have you ever used mentally handicapped to study an experimental vaccine?

A: What I'm saying is I don't recall specifically having done that, but that in the 1960s, it was not unusual to do that. And I wouldn't deny that I may have done so. (Discussion off the stenographic record.) BY MR. SIRI:

Q: I'm going to read you a sentence from what what's been previously marked as -.

MS. RUBY: No, that wasn't .

BY MR. SIRI:

Q: -- Exhibit 7.

MS. RUBY: That's not what got marked as Exhibit 7. That got -- the task force was seven.

MR. SIRI: Oh.

MS. NIEUSMA: So this should be 42.

MR. SIRI: Got it. Got it. Got it.

(Exhibit Plaintiff-42 was marked for identification.)

BY MR. SIRI:
Q: Well, in any event, you're not denying that you, that you -- well, there's an article entitled "Attenuation of RA 27/3 Rubella Virus in WI-38 Human Diploid Cells." Are you familiar with that article?
A: Yes.
Q: In that article, one of the things it says is 13 -- is one of the things it says is: 13 seroneg-ative mentally retarded children were given RA 27/3 vaccine?
A: Okay. Well, then that's, in that case that's what I did.
Q: Have you ever expressed that it's better to perform experiments on those less likely to be able to contribute to society, such as children with handicap, than with children with-out or adults without handicaps?
A: I don't remember specifically, but it's possible. And, again, I repeat that in the 1960s, that was more or less common practice. I've since changed my mind. But those were, that was a long time ago.
Q: Do you remember ever writing to the editor of "Ethics on Human Experimentation"?
A: I don't remember specifically, but I may well have.
Q: We'll mark this.

(Exhibit Plaintiff-43 was marked for identification.)

BY MR. SIRI:
Q: I'm going to hand you what's been marked as Exhibit 43. Do you recognize this letter you wrote to the editor?
A: Yes.
Q: Did you write this letter?
A: Yes.
Q: Is one of the things you wrote: The question is whether we are to have experiments performed on fully functioning adults and on children who are potentially contributors to society or to perform initial studies in children and adults who are human in form but not in social potential?
A: Yes.
Q: It may be objected that this question implies a Nazi philosophy, but I do not think that it is difficult to distinguish nonfunctioning persons from members of ethnic, racial, economic, or other groups.
A: Mm-hmm.
Q: Have you ever used babies of mothers in prison to study an experimental vaccine?
A: Yes.
Q: Have you ever used individuals under colonial rule to study an experimental vaccine?
A: Yes.
Q: Did you do so in the Belgian Congo?
A: Yes.
Q: Did that experiment involve almost a million people?
A: Well -- well, all right, yes.
Q: Did you ever visit what was the Belgian Congo and Ruanda-Urundi?
A: Yes.

Q: How many times?
A: Once.
MS. RUBY: Spell it.
MR. SIRI: R-U-A-N-D-A, dash, U-R-U-N-D-I .
BY MR. SIRI:
Q: When was that visit?
A: 1959.
Q: And how long were you there?
A: Oh, couple of months.
Q: Two months?
A: I think so, yes.
Q: Could it have been longer?
A: No. I don't think it was longer than that.
Q: What places did you visit?
A: What was then called Leopoldville, Stanleyville, Kivu.
Q: Kivu?
A: Yes.
Q: K-I-V-U?
A: Yes. Burundi.
MS. RUBY: Ms. Nieusma, are you back?
MS. NIEUSMA: I am.
THE WITNESS: Could have been a couple of other places, but I don't remember .
BY MR. SIRI:
Q: I've heard you talk, I've heard some of your, in some of your speeches you remembered this trip fondly, right?
A: Well, "fondly" may not be the right word, but I do remember it as an important event.
Q: In what order did you visit the places you just told me? Which one do you think visited first?
A: Leopoldville.
Q: Okay. And then after that?
A: Stanleyville.
Q: Then?
A: Then the eastern part of the Congo.
Q: Is that Kivu?
A: Yeah. And Bukavu. Bukavu.
MS. RUBY: Can you spell it? BY MR. SIRI:
Q: Is that before or after Burundi?
A: Before.
MS. RUBY: Can you spell those? BY MR. SIRI:
Q: Can you spell Bukavu.
A: B-U-K-A-V-U.
Q: So Leopoldville, then Stanleyville, then
Kivu, Bukum [sic], and then Burundi. So how long were you in Leopoldville?
A: Oh, gosh, I don't, I can't answer that question. I don't remember.
Q: Approximately.
A: A couple of weeks probably.
Q: How long in Stanleyville?

A: I don't know. Three, four weeks. I can't possibly remember that far back.

Q: And then how long in Kivu approximately?

A: Oh, a short time.

Q: And then Bakum [sic]?

A: I'm sorry?

Q: Bukum [sic]?

A: Oh, Bukavu?

Q: Bukavu.

COURT REPORTER: I don't know. The pronunciations are not matching the spellings, so I don't know what you're saying.

MR. SIRI: Sorry .

BY MR. SIRI:

Q: B-U-K-U-V -.

A: B-U-K-A-V-U.

Q: K-A-V-U. Sorry. Bukavu, approximately how long?

A: Couple of days.

Q: Okay. And then finally Burundi?

A: Again, I don't know. Maybe a week. I'm not sure.

Q: Okay. What were you doing in Leopoldville?

A: I was examining the data on oral polio vaccination in the city.

Q: Anything else?

A: No.

Q: Did you vaccinate anybody?

A: Personally, no.

Q: How about in, what were you doing in Stanleyville?

A: I was visiting the chimpanzee laboratory and talking to scientists in Stanleyville.

Q: Talking about what?

A: Well, about polio mainly.

Q: And what about polio?

A: What about polio? Obviously, they were having polio, and we were talking about how to protect the people against polio.

Q: And did you the vaccinate anybody while you were in Stanleyville personally?

A: Personally, no.

Q: What did you do in Kivu?

A: As I recall, I just visited the place.

Q: Any purpose?

A: I don't think so, no.

Q: Did you vaccinate anybody personally?

A: It was a scenic area.

Q: Did you vaccinate anybody personally there?

A: No.

Q: What about Bukavu?

A: I did not do any vaccination there either.

Q: What were you doing there?

A: I was just visiting.

Q: Like a tourist?

A: Yes.

Q: Same thing with Kivu, as a tourist?
A: Yes.
Q: What about Burundi?
A: There, I had some discussions with scientists.
Q: About what?
A: About polio.
Q: Okay. Did you, other than that, did you do anything else in Burundi?
A: No.
Q: Did you vaccinate anybody personally?
A: No.
Q: Okay. During your entire trip, did you vaccinate anybody personally?
A: No.
Q: So your whole trip to Belgian Congo and Ruanda-Urundi, you never vaccinated anybody personally?
A: That is correct. I also stopped in Kikwit, which was to observe a vaccination campaign.
Q: That was between what cities?
A: Well, geographically it's between Leopoldville and Stanleyville. I don't recall in what order I visited it.
Q: You don't know if it was before or after Stanleyville?
A: No, I don't.
Q: How long were you in Kikwit?
A: Well, just a day or two.
Q: That was just to observe a -.
A: Vaccination campaign.
Q: -- campaign. Did you observe a vaccination campaign in any of the other cities?
A: Stanleyville probably. Leopoldville was, as I said before, to collect data from prior vaccination.
Q: What were you doing in Ruanda-Urundi?
A: Talking to people.
Q: Again, about polio vaccine?
A: Yes.
Q: But not vaccinating anybody?
A: No.
Q: Not part of any vaccination campaign there either?
A: No.
Q: Do you believe that someone can have a valid religious objection to refusing a vaccine?
A: No.
Q: Do you take issue with religious beliefs?
A: Yes.
Q: You have said that, quote: Vaccination is always under attack by religious zealots who believe that the will of God includes death and disease?
A: Yes.
Q: You stand by that statement?
A: I absolutely do.
Q: Are you an atheist?
A: Yes.
Q: Do you accept that some people hold religious beliefs that are inherently unprovable?

A: Yes, I'm sure they do.

Q: You said that, quote: Vaccination is always under attack by a legal system that profits from the failure of most people to understand risk/benefit ratios or public health issues, correct?

A: Yes.

Q: Can you explain what you mean by that, shortly?

A: I mean that the risk from vaccines, for example, is considerably less than the risk from disease, but people don't necessarily understand that. It's similar to the situation where people may not fly, but they're willing to drive in cars where the risks are much higher. And what was the second point about?

Q: Public health issues.

A: Public health issues, yes. Not understanding the importance of high vaccination coverage in prevention of disease.

Q: One child can make a difference?

A: One child probably doesn't make a difference, but a collection of one childs do make a difference.

Q: At the most recent ACIP meeting, you spoke and gave ACIP three pieces of advice, correct?

A: Yes.

Q: One of them was to conduct more vaccine safety studies to prove the anti-vaccinationists wrong, right?

A: Yes. Correct.

Q: Okay. If the science to prove vaccines safe already exist, why would more safety studies be needed to prove the anti-vaccinationists wrong?

A: Because there are so many people, as you can see on the web, who have these beliefs about vaccines. And as we have discussed throughout this long day, it would be valuable to have more safety data.

Q: Like a vaccinated versus unvaccinated study, correct?

A: If such a study is feasible.

Q: Shouldn't vaccine safety studies be done for the sake of making vaccines safer, not for the purpose and with the pre-determined objective of proving so-called anti-vaccinationists wrong?

A: Well, absolutely. I do not deny that there are known reactions to vaccines. Fortunately, they rarely are serious. I support more research on every aspect of vaccines.

Q: And your claim that they're rarely serious is from your book, right?

A: Yes.

Q: Okay. When is the last time that you received a vaccine, Dr. Plotkin?

A: Zoster -- oh, no. Influenza vaccine actually, not more than several weeks ago.

Q: Do you get the flu shot every year?

A: Yes.

Q: Have you ever missed a year?

A: No.

Q: Have you received the zoster vaccine? It sounds like you have.

A: Yes.

Q: Zoster, Z-O-S-T-E-R. When did you receive that?

A: I've received now two doses, and I'm looking forward to receiving the new Zoster vaccine as soon as I can buy it.

Q: Have you received a PCV13 vaccine?

A: Yes.

Q: Have you received a PPSV23 vaccine?

A: Yes.

Q: Hep B vaccine?

A: Yes.

Q: Let me do that again. Have you received a hep B vaccine?

A: Yes.

Q: Have you received a hepatitis A vaccine?

A: Yes.

Q: Have you received a MenACWY or MPSV4 vaccine?

A: I believe so. That was a long time in the past because those vaccines have been available for a long time. I have to check my records. But I think particularly when I traveled to the Africa, I believe I took it.

Q: Have you received a MenB vaccine?

A: Not yet, no.

Q: Have you received a Hib vaccine?

A: Oh, Hib. I was long past the age of Hib when it was developed.

Q: When is the last time you got a tetanus/diphtheria-containing vaccine?

A: Within the last ten years. I don't remember exactly when, but -.

Q: Do you think all adults should be required to receive all vaccines on the CDC's adult immunization schedule?

A: That's somewhat of a difficult question because adults, of course, have the ability to make their own decisions. Tetanus is, is a vaccine that, how shall I put it? I guess it's a choice whether you're willing to be susceptible to tetanus or not. For pertussis, I think there's increasing reason that, to say that all adults should be vaccinated against pertussis. So it's, let's say, let's say, open to discussion at this point for DTaP anyway.

Q: You'd support a law that would require adults to get the DTaP?

A: At this point, 2017 [sic], I wouldn't insist on that for all adults. I would insist on it for children and adolescents. But the data, the reason I say that is because the data showing protection against pertussis in older adults is really not that solid, not that available.

Q: Did you ever experience an adverse vaccine reaction?

A: Personally.

Q: Yes.

A: No.

Q: Have you ever witnessed someone experience an adverse vaccine reaction?

A: I've witnessed people fainting after vaccination.

Q: Anything else?

A: Certainly I've seen people complain of pain at the injection site. And in the rubella days, women complaining of joint pains after vaccination. I think that's it.

Q: When you say "fainting," after what vaccine was that?

A: Oh, actually that was, that was tetanus, as I recall. It was a high school athlete.

Q: Do you know anyone that's experienced a serious adverse reaction -.

A: Personally, no.

Q: Did your grandchildren receive the hepatitis B vaccine on the first day of life as recommended by the CDC?

A: Of course.

(Reporter clarification.)

Q: Have your grandchildren received the hepatitis B vaccine on the first day of life as recommended by the CDC?

A: Yes.

Q: Do you think there's a safe threshold of how many vaccines can be administered at one time?

A: My answer to that is I don't know. I don't think there's any evidence that the six that are currently generally given together is a problem. So I don't know if eventually there's some theoretical threshold, but I am not aware of any evidence for that yet.

Q: Okay. But before you would say, for example, getting 30 vaccines in one day was safe, you'd probably want to get the data to support it?

A: Yes.

Q: That data doesn't yet exist obviously, right?

A: No.

Q: Do you intend to appear at trial in this matter to testify?

A: No, I do not.

Q: Do you intend to appear via video conference to testify in this trial in this case?

A: Well, I haven't been asked. I suppose I might consider a video conference. But no one has asked me. And I'm not, I would say, very inclined to do that. And you know, while we're on tape, so to speak, I want to stipulate, since you were so interested in my income, that I am doing this pro bono.

Q: But as you sit here today, you're still receiving remuneration from all four major vaccine makers, correct?

A: Yes.

Q: And from -- so getting close to the end. I don't have much left. A few more. There was a controversy revolving around the origin of AIDS and the OPV vaccine, correct?

A: Yes.

Q: You disputed any connection between OPV vaccine and AIDS in two papers submitted to the Royal Society in which you stated, quote: There was no gun, the chimpanzees; no bullet, the virus; no shooter, the manufacturer of the vaccine chimpanzee cells; and no motive to use chimp cells or to hide the fact, correct?

A: Yeah. I also said the only smoke was created by Mr. Hooper.

Q: Right. Who is that?

A: He's a British journalist, which puts him at the lower end of journalism.

MR. SIRI: Mark this.

(Exhibit Plaintiff-44 was marked for identification.)

BY MR. SIRI:

Q: Dr. Plotkin, I'm going to hand you what's been marked as Plaintiff's Exhibit 44. And I'm also going to hand you what's been marked as Plaintiff's Exhibit 45.

(Exhibit Plaintiff-45 was marked for identification.)

BY MR. SIRI:

Q: Are these the two papers that you submitted to the Royal Society -.

A: Yes.

Q: -- disputing -- one second, please. -- disputing any connection between OPV vaccine and AIDS -.

A: Yes.

Q: -- correct? Is everything that you wrote in these two articles -- strike that. Is everything written in the two articles, Royal Society articles that you submitted, which are marked as Exhibits 44 and 45, true?

A: Well, I certainly hope so.

Q: Is that -- I'm sorry, Dr. Plotkin. Is that yes?

A: Yes. Yes. And I should also add that my conclusions have been verified by other scientists who now have shown that HIV originated in the 1920s in Cameroon.

Q: At the end of -- Dr. Plotkin, at the end of Exhibit 44, the article entitled "Untruths and Consequences," you state that -- strike that. I apologize. I'm sorry, Dr. Plotkin. Can you look at Exhibit 45. I'm sorry. The end of Exhibit 45, it states that letters cited in this paper will be deposited in the library of the College of Physicians of Philadelphia or the University of Leuven, L-E-U-V-E-N, correct?

A: Yes.

Q: Have you deposited those letters and papers?

A: I have, yes.

Q: Okay. When did you deposit all of those letters and papers?

A: Oh, gosh, probably at least five years ago now.

Q: So all of the letters cited in this document are, have been deposited in where?

A: The College of Physicians of Philadelphia.

Q: And they're in possession of all of the letters cited in this document?

A: Well, I believe so. I have to go over the list. But that certainly was my intention, and I believe I have done so.

Q: Is that publicly available at the University of Philadelphia?

A: It's a good question. I imagine so. I deposited them there basically so that they could be examined after I'm dead, but -.

Q: Yeah.

A: -- I don't know. I've never been asked.

Q: If they're not publicly available, would you provide copies?

A: Well, I have to ask the College of Physicians to do that.

Q: Would you authorize them to release copies?

A: I'd authorize them, sure.

Q: Okay. If you could please take a look at the -.

A: I'm not sure why you're asking the question. Are you -.

Q: I'm asking the question -.

A: -- accusing me of launching AIDS? Or what is the point?

Q: Absolutely not, Dr. Plotkin. You made a promise in here to deposit papers, and I'm purely asking you if you made that, fulfilled that promise. That's it.

A: Yes, I did.

Q: That's all. I'm not accusing you of anything. And in the other paper entitled "Untruths and Consequences," in the second paragraph, it says: The evidence I present is based on papers and documents of the time from my personal files.

A: Mm-hmm.

Q: Have those also been deposited in the library of Philadelphia?

A: No. Certainly not all of them. I have extensive files. I don't throw anything out.

Q: You still have all of those?

A: Yes.

Q: I assume you don't have an issue sharing copies of those?

A: No. My wife would love to get rid of all of them. But I don't...

Q: So you've said that the AIDS/OPV hypothesis has been disproven, correct?

A: Yes.

Q: A few quick questions. Just approximately how many human samples that predate 1959 have been tested for HIV?

A: That predate 1959? I don't know that there are any such samples available. The first samples that I recall being available were from 1960, and they had already some HIV seropositive individuals. But that was in Leopoldville. They were individuals who had not received the oral polio vaccine.

Q: So -- but in terms of samples that predate 1959, have there been any such samples tested for HIV?

A: I have to think about that. I -- oh, well, there have been samples from elsewhere in the world; but from the Belgian Congo -.

Q: Yeah.

A: -- I don't think that any such samples have been available.

Q: Are you aware of whether there currently exists any samples of polio vaccine that was in the Belgian Congo at any time between 1959 and 1960?

A: Whether the Wistar has kept them or not, I don't know. Fortunately, at the time of the Royal Society, I was able to go to Wistar and find specimens that had been used in the Congo or from the same lot that had been used in the Congo. But whether that still exists or not, I have no idea.

Q: Well, I'm curious as just, is there any samples that were actually in the Belgian Congo that have been, that you're aware of?

A: That were tested?

Q: That were tested.

A: I don't, really don't know the answer to that question. The vaccine that was used, the oral polio vaccine that was used, I believe was entirely used up in the vaccination campaign. So I don't think it's likely that material used in the vaccination campaign was repatriated. But fortunately, we had material from the same lots that were used in the Congo. And that had been retained at the Wistar.

Q: But as far as you're aware, in terms of actual samples, a sample that was actually in the Belgian Congo, you're not -- are you saying you're not aware of any such sample?

A: No, I am not aware of any such sample.

Q: Do you know if any such sample ever -- are you aware of any such sample that existed after 1960?

A: I don't -- I'm not aware that anything existed.

Q: So are you familiar with an article entitled "Vaccination with the CHAT Strain of Type 1 Attenuated Poliomyelitis Virus in Leopoldville, Belgian Congo"?

A: Yes.

Q: Okay. In the article -- you're one of the authors of the article?

A: Yes.

Q: So on page 2 of this article, it states: The titer of the vaccine after a day's use was checked periodically by sending frozen aliquots -.

A: Aliquots, yes.

Q: -- thank you, aliquots, A-L-I-Q-U-O-T-S, to the Wistar Institute, Philadelphia, Pennsylvania, USA?

A: Yes.

Q: What does that mean?

A: Well, it means that in order to be sure that the vaccine used still contained enough virus, they sent back samples to be titered for the quantity of virus.

Q: So they sent back samples of the oral polio -.

A: Yes.

Q: -- being used -.

A: Yes.

Q: -- in the Belgian Congo?

A: Yes.

Q: And they did that periodically?

A: Yes.

Q: But to your knowledge, none of those survived after 1960?

A: No. I think they were tested and then discarded. I mean, they, aside from legal value, they would have had no value because they were used; they could not ever be used again. So they would have been discarded.

Q: It would be helpful for you if some of those were saved, right?

A: It would have been, yes. But at the time nobody thought about that.

Q: If any, if such a sample were to have survived someplace on the planet, where would you think that would be?

A: Difficult to say. I mean, the laboratory in Stanleyville no longer exists. I have no idea where it could be. No.

Q: Do you think such a sample will ever be located?

A: I doubt it.

Q: Last question on this topic and we'll move on. Did you or any of your Wistar colleagues ever carry any human cells, such as WISH or WI-1, or polio vaccines grown in such human cells to the Belgian Congo?

A: No. At least I certainly have not.

Q: Are you aware of any such -.

A: No, I am not aware.

Q: -- vaccines being -.

A: No, I'm not aware of those cells being carried to the Congo. If they had been, it would have been for experimental purposes, certainly not for vaccination purposes.

Q: So you're not aware of them being carried or used there, right?

A: Not that I'm aware of, no.

Q: Isn't it true that in 2014, the FDA announced, quote: Although individuals immunized with an acellular pertussis vaccine may be protected from disease, they may still become infected with the bacteria without always getting sick and are able to spread infection to others, end quote?

A: Yes. That's on the basis of the studies in baboons.

Q: That's the Warfel study?

A: Yes.

Q: We discussed earlier that the baboons are the -- would probably be the best surrogates for humans, right?

A: Yes.

Q: Because you couldn't ethically expose humans to pertussis, correct?

A: Yes.

Q: So the Warfel studies would be the best evidence -- would the Warfel studies, the one in 2014 and 2016, which were conducted by the FDA, correct?

A: Yes.

Q: Those would be the best evidence as to the ability, as to whether or not acellular pertussis vaccine prevented infection and transmission of pertussis, correct?

A: Yes.

Q: And I think we talked about this earlier. In your estimation, what percent of adults would you say are actually immune to pertussis?

A: It's a very good question, and I don't know the answer to that because immunity to pertussis is complex. And so just measuring serum wouldn't necessarily give you a firm idea as to what percentage of adults are immune. But judging from the frequency of pertussis in adults, I don't think the immunity level is very high, because clearly adults are getting pertussis.

Q: Could you estimate what percentage of the adult population in the United States you think is immune to pertussis?

A: Immune? Well, I think probably 50, 60 percent could be immune. But it's difficult because immunity wanes.

Q: Right.

A: So they may, people become susceptible again. And as I said now twice, there is a lot of pertussis in adults. That's been shown. So a significant proportion of adults are susceptible and not immune.

Q: Fifty to 60 percent is your highest estimation -.

A: Yes.

Q: -- it sounded like, right?

A: Yes.

Q: No more than that? A I don't think so.

Q: Okay. The diphtheria vaccine creates antibodies only to a toxin released by the diphtheria bacteria, correct?

A: Correct.

Q: It doesn't create any antibodies to the actual diphtheria bacteria itself?

A: Yes, that's true. But it is also true, certainly appears to be true, that if the organism can't produce a toxin, it has a great difficulty in surviving. And so the observation is that where the vaccine is used, the organism disappears. So it's very difficult to find it in the U.S., for example. But in Russia where vaccination has not been always complete, there are still cases of diphtheria.

Q: Can you, how do you define anti-vaccinationists or anti-vaxxers, as you've used them here today?

A: How do I define them?

Q: Yeah. What does that mean to you? You use those terms, and I'm just, I'm actually not exactly sure what you mean by that.

A: People opposed to vaccination for a variety of reasons, some of which are based on false inferences from scientific data.

Q: If somebody were opposed to vaccines because they believed there was insufficient data for them to make a decision about the actual risks, not the benefits, but the risks, would you consider that person an anti-vaxxer?

A: If they refused to be vaccinated themselves or refused to have their children vaccinated, I would call them an anti-vaccination person, yes.

Q: Is there anybody who could refuse a vaccine who you would not label anti-vaxxer?

A: Yes. If there are individuals who are immunosuppressed, for example, and, therefore, have a contraindication to certain vaccines, that to me would be a reasonable decision on their part.

Q: But, otherwise, you believe that anybody else who refuses a vaccine is doing so based on misinformation?

A: Generally speaking, yes. Now, as I said before, I can imagine an adult deciding that they don't want the advantages of vaccination out of, for whatever reason. I think the situation for children is quite different because one is making a decision for somebody else and also making a decision that has important implications for public health.

Q: So in the case of an adult, you think it's okay for the adult to make a decision for themselves to take on a risk, even though it could implicate public health, but not the case for a child?

A: No. It depends. For example, if you're a healthcare worker and you refuse to be vaccinated against diseases that you could potentially transmit to patients, I don't think you should have the option of making that decision.

Q: Earlier we discussed that there hasn't been a wild case of polio in the United States since 1979, correct?

A: Right.

Q: The United States currently only uses inactivated polio vaccine, correct?

A: Yes.

Q: The United States does not use oral polio vaccine, correct?

A: Correct.

Q: If there were an outbreak of polio in the United States -.

A: Yes.

Q: -- isn't it true that we would have to, that we would have to return to using oral polio vaccine to stop the spread of polio in the United States?

A: It might well be the case; however, individuals who have received the inactivated vaccines will not themselves get polio. They may get infected and transmit to others, which is one of the reasons why one might resort to OPV. But the individual himself would not be susceptible.

Q: Is that because the IPV creates IGG antibodies in the blood towards -.

A: Yes.

Q: But it doesn't create IGA immunity in the intestinal tract?

A: Correct.

Q: And it is in the intestinal tract where the polio virus multiplies, correct?

A: Yes.

Q: So a person vaccinated with IPV can still become infected and transmit polio virus, correct?

A: Yes, although in point of fact, IPV does protect the nasopharynx. So in this country where hygiene and sewage, et cetera, are good, the possibility of transmitting from an IPV vaccinee is much less than it is, let's say, in Africa where sewage contamination is great.

Q: When you say nasopharynx, what is that?

A: The throat.

Q: So you're saying IPV does create immunity within the throat?

A: Yes.

Q: There are studies that show that?

A: Yes, absolutely.

Q: Okay. How do those studies make that determination?

A: Well, by culturing people who are exposed to polio, who have had IPV, and also by showing that antibody diffuses into the throat much better than it does into the gut.

Q: In the Warfel study -- I'm sorry. Strike that. Do you know the names of those studies, by any chance?

A: Gosh, again, they're in the book.

Q: Are they in your book?

A: Yes, absolutely.

Q: Okay. And in terms of efficacy, does IPV vaccination as -- in childhood last a lifetime?

A: You know, that's an interesting question, and I think the answer is yes. Studies that have been done have shown quite good persistence of antibody after IPV. Now, does it last forever? I can't say that, but certainly lasts a long time.

Q: How about 30 years after vaccination; what do you think the efficacy is approximately?

A: I would just be totally speculating, but I think most people would still be protected because you don't need much antibody against polio to be protected. Levels of dilutions of one to four, one to eight are probably protective.

Q: But you're not sure?

A: I'm not sure about 30 years. I'm sure about the levels that are protective.

Q: Thirty years, you're not sure about what percent of the people vaccinated are still immune to polio?

A: No. But I do know that that persistence is good and that the likelihood is that most people, even 30 years, will still be protected.

Q: Forty years?

A: I can't really guess any more than that.

Q: The data doesn't exist?

A: No. I don't believe they exist.

Q: Well, what do you estimate is the current efficacy of the mumps vaccine shortly after vaccination?

A: Oh, shortly after vaccination, there's no doubt that the efficacy is high. It's 80, 90 percent. And after two doses, immediately after two doses, the efficacy is very high. Unfortunately, the efficacy diminishes with time, and that has caused a problem in universities that have outbreaks of mumps because the college kids are -.

Q: No longer immune?

A: -- intimately associated. Yes. Although the efficacy even then is probably in the order of 70, 80 percent.

Q: 70, 80 percent. What about, what about 30 years after vaccination; what's the efficacy?

A: I have no idea.

Q: Twenty years?

A: I don't think studies have been done more than ten years after vaccine.

Q: What do you estimate is the current efficacy of the rubella vaccine ten years after vaccination?

A: Based on the data that are available, it is very high. The so-called B cell memory after rubella vaccine, I'm happy to say, is very good.

Q: How about 20 years?

A: I think it will still be present.

Q: Thirty years?

A: I think so.

Q: High efficacy still, you think?

A: I think so.

Q: But no study has been done?

A: Actually, there are studies, at least 20-year studies. I'm not sure about 30, but immunity is very long-lasting.

Q: And -- okay. And the studies would be in your book?

A: Yes.

Q: What would you estimate is the current efficacy of the measles vaccine 20 years after vaccination?

A: Well, again, it appears to be quite good. Twenty years, again, I'm, don't have it in my head as a study done 20 years later. But certainly studies done sometime after vaccination have shown good persistence of antibodies. And once again, you don't need a whole lot of antibody to prevent you from getting measles.

Q: Do you know a percentage?

A: Of?

Q: Of people that are still immune 20 years out from the measles vaccine?

A: Not off the top of my head, but I feel relatively sure that it's quite high.

Q: Is it important to get a tetanus vaccine?

A: Well, it's important if you don't want to get tetanus, yes.

Q: The tetanus vaccine was introduced into routine child schedule in the late 1940s, correct?

A: Yes.

Q: When the tetanus vaccine was introduced there were only about four cases of tetanus per million people, correct?

A: If you say so. I don't remember.

Q: Are you familiar with what, the CDC Pink Book?

A: Yes.

Q: If the CDC Pink Book said that it was four cases of tetanus per million, would you dispute that?

A: I'll accept that.

Q: You do accept that. And that's just the number of cases, not deaths, right?

A: Yes.

Q: And you think it's a public health imperative for people to be vaccinated against tetanus, correct?

A: I think it's the wise thing to do if you don't want to be under risk of getting tetanus if you have an injury.

Q: To prevent something that was a few cases in a million, correct?

A: Yes. But a deadly disease.

Q: Do we know whether the tetanus vaccine causes more or less than a few cases of serious adverse reactions after vaccination?

A: I don't believe it causes a whole lot of serious reactions, no.

Q: I'm going to show you what's -.

MS. NIEUSMA: Do you know how much longer we have to go? Just so I have an idea.

MR. SIRI: Yeah, sure. I think that we've only got about 15 more minutes.

VIDEO OPERATOR: That's exactly how much we have left on the tape.

MS. NIEUSMA: Very good.

MR. SIRI: We're almost done.

(Exhibit Plaintiff-46 was marked for identification.)

BY MR. SIRI:

Q: The CDC and FDA maintained something called the Vaccine Adverse Events Reporting System, correct?

A: Yes.

Q: And that's where anybody, including doctors, can go and report what they believe to be an adverse reaction from a vaccine -.

A: Right.

Q: -- right?

A: Correct.

Q: There's no, anybody can submit a report, right?

A: That's correct.

Q: Okay. And the FDA and CDC compiled that data and make it available online, correct?

A: Yes.

Q: Okay. I'm going hand you a, what's been marked as Plaintiff's Exhibit 46. Okay? And this is a printout of the VAERS data for all adverse reactions reported to tetanus-containing vaccines in the last ten years. If you take a look, do you see that in the last ten years, there have been 985 deaths reported -.

A: Yes.

Q: -- to have followed any tetanus-containing vaccine?

A: Yes.

Q: That would average to about 98.5 reports of death per year -.

A: Yes.

Q: -- over the last ten years. Okay. And there's also 23,981 emergency room or office visits after tetanus-containing vaccine in the last ten years?

A: Yes.

Q: And it also lists, last one, 1,256 permanent disabilities reported after tetanus-containing vaccine in the last ten years, correct?

A: Yeah.

Q: That would be about an average of 125 per year, right?

A: Yes.

Q: So, but we don't, because these are just reports and not done in some kind of randomized, controlled study, we don't actually know whether or not the tetanus vaccine is causing these deaths and permanent disabilities, correct?

A: Correct.

Q: Okay. But it's possible it could be, correct?

A: It's, anything is possible, yes.

Q: Don't you think a study should be done to determine -- strike that. Strike that. Isn't it true that VAERS only receives a tiny fraction of the reportable adverse events after vaccination?

A: Well, I can't give you a percentage, but all physicians are asked to report putative reactions to the VAERS system. So I don't think the VAERS system covers a tiny portion of alleged reactions. I think, rather, probably most are reported. But I, I cannot confirm that.

(Exhibit Plaintiff-47 was marked for identification.)

BY MR. SIRI:

Q: Dr. Plotkin, I'm going to show you what's been marked as Plaintiff's Exhibit 47. This is a report entitled "Electronic Support for Public Health - Vaccine Adverse Events Reporting System," correct? Let me know when you're ready, Dr. Plotkin.

A: I'm ready.

Q: The title of this report, Dr. Plotkin, is "Electronic Support for Public Health - Vaccine Adverse Event Reporting System," correct?

A: Yes.

Q: And this was a study conducted by Harvard Medical School and the Harvard Pilgrim Healthcare, correct?

A: Yes.

Q: And it was are done via a grant from an agency within HHS, correct?

A: Yes.

Q: And the purpose of this study was to attempt to automate VAERS reporting?

A: Yes.

Q: The reason that Harvard did this study and the reason that HHS paid for it, if you look at page 6 -.

A: Yes.

Q: -- do you see where it says: Fewer than 1 -- it's right in the middle paragraph: Fewer than 1 percent of vaccine adverse events are reported?

A: Well, yes, I see the statement. I don't see the reference, but...

Q: Let's take a look at the results of that study, then. If you go to the first sentence of the page that you're on right now -.

A: Yeah.

Q: -- where it says "results," isn't it true that it says: Preliminary data were collected from June 2006 through October 2009 on 715 -- 715,000 patients?

A: Yes.

Q: And 1.4 million doses of 45 different vaccines were given to 376,452 individuals?

A: Yes.

Q: So about 376,000 individuals received a vaccine, correct?

A: Yes.

Q: Out of these doses, 35,570 possible reactions were identified, correct?

A: Yes.

Q: So out of 376,000 people that received vaccines, they identified 35,570 possible reactions, right?

A: Yes.

Q: And now -.

A: Well, it's out of 1.4 million, which is 2.6 percent.

Q: Doses, correct?

A: Yes.

Q: Meaning maybe some individuals had -.

A: More than one vaccine.

Q: And had reactions at different times to different vaccines, right?

A: Yes.

Q: Maybe some people were more susceptible to a vaccine reaction, and so they got, had a reaction every time they had a vaccine, right?

A: Well, we don't know that.

Q: We don't know. Assuming that each individual only had one vaccine reaction, then 10 percent of the individuals would have had a vaccine reaction?

A: Mm-hmm. Yes.

Q: All right. So, now, at the beginning of this study, the CDC was cooperating with these grant participants, correct -- grant recipients, correct?

A: Yes.

Q: And they helped define what is an adverse reaction, right?

A: Yes.

Q: And they helped define the algorithms to use, right?

A: Yes.

Q: And they also helped to define what reports should be excluded, correct?

A: I guess so.

Q: What events, I'm sorry, should be excluded from being considered, you know, report-able, right?

A: Yes.

Q: After, however, they collected this data and they generated these 35,000 reports, they then wanted to submit those reports to VAERS and automate it so that those reports could continue to be submitted, correct?

A: Yes.

Q: correct? But the CDC wouldn't cooperate with them,

A: or not. Well, I have no idea whether that's true

Q: On page 5, Dr. Plotkin, at the end of the second paragraph, it says: Real -- does it say: Real data transmission of nonphysician-approved reports to the CDC were unable to commence by the end of this -- as by the end of this project, the CDC had yet to respond to multiple requests to partner for this activity? Is that what it says?

A: That's what it says.

Q: Okay. So, and this study says that less than 1 percent of adverse events are reported to VAERS, right?

A: Well, I have to check that, but I think that's correct.

Q: Okay. Are you aware that there are other, other governmental reports that make similar estimates for VAERS?

A: I'm aware that not everything is reported to VAERS, yes.

Q: Are you aware that governmental reports show that, that governmental reports like this one show that the rate of reporting to VAERS is extremely low, and in this instance they say Harvard said less than 1 percent?

A: Yes, apparently, yes. However, it has to be reminded that reporting to VAERS is sup-posed to occur whether or not you think there's been a reaction. So whether or not the reactions are true or not is not something that VAERS decides.

Q: Right. But let's just assume for a second here, so if, let's go back to what's been marked as Exhibit 46, okay? Let's assume that a full 1 percent of associated adverse events are re-ported; wouldn't that take the number of deaths to 98,000, then, that were associated with the vaccine?

A: I think it's likely the deaths are reported more often than trivial reactions. So I wouldn't be able to extrapolate from that number.

Q: Right.

A: But, you know, obviously death is more dramatic.

Q: Let me show you, I think, one final exhibit.

VIDEO OPERATOR: We have six minutes left on the disc .

BY MR. SIRI:

Q: I'm going to hand you what's been marked as Plaintiff's Exhibit 48.

(Exhibit Plaintiff-48 was marked for identification.)

BY MR. SIRI:

Q: This is the VAERS report for all adverse events for all vaccines just since January of 2016. Do you see that?

A: Yes.

Q: If this -.

A: My wife is getting upset.

Q: Well, don't tell her you offered her up for a deposition. If this represents even 3 percent or 5 percent of reported events, doesn't this concern you in that maybe it really indicates -- strike that. It reports 751 life-threatening reactions, correct?

A: Yes.

Q: And that's only since January of 2016, correct?

A: Yes.

Q: If that's only, if that's a full 1 percent, then that would be 75,000 life-threatening reactions that would have been reported, correct?

A: That's the arithmetic, yes.

Q: That's the kind of event that would happen pretty soon after vaccination, correct?

A: Well, events that happen after vaccination, yes -.

Q: Okay.

A: -- but not necessarily because of vaccination.

Q: But until a properly controlled saline placebo study is actually done or -- strike that. Until we compare the total health outcomes -- strike that. Would you support a study that compared total health outcomes between vaccinated and unvaccinated children, Dr. Plotkin?

A: Will I support such a study? Yes. If the protocol was scientifically valid, yes, I would support such a study. I don't really put much faith into the VAERS system for a number of reasons, some of which you've cited. I take much more, I put much more confidence in the vaccine safety data, data which are better controlled and which come from institutions that see large numbers of patients.

Q: Would you work to support such a study?

A: Again, if such a study were scientifically feasible, I would support it, yes.

Q: Don't you want to know what the results of that study show?

A: If the study is done, yes, of course.

Q: In terms of the Vaccine Safety Datalink which you just mentioned, that's not available to the public, correct?

A: I think they publicly report in the scientific literature -.

Q: If independent researchers want to get access to the VSD while -.

A: I, I don't know what the circumstances are regarding access to data.

Q: Well, then I won't -.

A: I simply don't know.

Q: I won't ask you questions about that, if you don't know it.

VIDEO OPERATOR: Two minutes.

MR. SIRI: Okay. Well, I am, I'm done with my questioning. And I will, if opposing counsel intends to ask any questions, then I reserve to ask some rebuttal questions as well. But, otherwise, I'm done with my questioning for today.

MS. NIEUSMA: You know what? If Dr. Plotkin is going to testify, I'm going to have him here in Michigan, so I'm not concerned about it. Let's just call it a day. Dr. Plotkin, I'll give you a call tomorrow if you're available for a quick phone call.

THE WITNESS: Actually, no. I'll be in A meeting in Philadelphia, but I will be available on Monday.

MS. NIEUSMA: Perfect. I will call you on Monday.

THE WITNESS: Okay.

COURT REPORTER: Counsel, don't hang up, please. Stanley Plotkin, M.D.

MS. NIEUSMA: All right.

VIDEO OPERATOR: This ends disc five. It concludes the deposition of Dr. Stanley Plotkin. We are going off the record. The time is 18:43. COURT REPORTER: Ms. Nieusma, do you need a copy of today's transcript?

MS. NIEUSMA: I do not.

COURT REPORTER: Is the witness going to read and sign?

MS. NIEUSMA: He certainly can. It's generally not something we do around here. But he can do it if anybody wants him to. (Discussion off the record.)

MR. SIRI: I'll talk to you after. (Witness excused.) (Deposition concluded at 6:42 p.m.)

www.ingramcontent.com/pod-product-compliance
Lightning Source LLC
Chambersburg PA
CBHW051025030426

42336CB00015B/2718